A Practical Manual for Topographical Anatomy in Dentistry

4th Edition

Practical manual for Dental and Dental Hygiene students for learning topographical anatomy of the head and neck region, thorax, abdomen, upper limb and neuroanatomy.

Successfully applied from 2006 to 2011 in University College Cork.

Ideal for designing a course in Dentistry by instructors and demonstrators.

Recommended to students to prepare themselves for the course and revise anatomy through self-directed learning.

Contains practical sessions with dissections schemes and gives an outline of prosections with explanations of anatomical terms and clinical links.

A Practical Manual for Topographical Anatomy in Dentistry

4th Edition

Deniz M. Yilmazer-Hanke, Dr. med. habil.
College Lecturer
Department of Anatomy
University College Cork
Ireland

Current address:
Associate Professor
Department of Biomedical Sciences
Creighton University
Omaha, Nebraska, U.S.A.

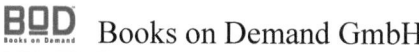 Books on Demand GmbH

Norderstedt

2011

Address of author:
Deniz Yilmazer-Hanke, Dr. med. habil.
Associate Professor
Department of Biomedical Sciences
Creighton University
2500 California Plaza
Omaha, NE 68178, U.S.A.

1st Edition   2007
2nd Edition   2008
3rd Edition   2010
4th Edition   2011

Yilmazer-Hanke, D.M. (Deniz M.)
A Practical Manual for Topographical Anatomy in Dentistry. 4th Edition.

Herstellung und Verlag (Production and Publisher):
Book on Demand GmbH, Norderstedt
AG Kiel | HRB 4551 NO | GF: Dr. M. Hagenmüller, H. Bellmann

Address of Publisher:
Book on Demand GmbH,
In de Tarpen 42,
D-22848 Norderstedt, Germany
phone   +49 40 - 53 43 35-11; fax   +49 40 - 53 43 35-84
email   info@bod.de; website www.bod.de

Bibliographische Information Der Deutschen Nationalbibliothek
Die Deutsche Bibliothek verzeichnet diese Publikation in der Deutschen Nationalbibliographie; detaillierte bibliographische Daten sind im Internet über http://dnb.d-nb.de abrufbar.

Printed in Germany

ISBN 9783842379497

CONTENTS

mucosa and lacrimal gland; Chorda tympani nerve from facial nerve (CN. VII) – Autonomic fibres to submandibular & sublingual glands, and sensation of taste; Lesser petrosal nerve (CN. IX) – Autonomic supply of the parotid gland

1. INTRODUCTION

1.1 TOPICS OF THE COURSE

This is a practical manual for teaching *Topographical Anatomy* to *Dental* and *Dental Hygiene Students*. It does not replace a textbook, e-book, atlas or glossary for learning anatomy.

The manual is recommended to *Instructors and Demonstrators* to design their practical sessions. It provides <u>Dissection Schemes</u> of the Head and Neck Region. In addition, the regions, which can be learned ideally by studying <u>Prosections</u>, are described. The prosections can be *prepared in advance* by Prosectors, and the structures can be labeled with *name tags* before the practical sessions. If the facilities allow for using *histology sections* or *slides*, these can also be included into the practical sessions (e.g. with the aid of microscopes or video monitors).

Students can use the manual to <u>prepare</u> themselves to the practical sessions, for <u>self-directed learning</u> purposes, and/or to <u>revise</u> their knowledge in topographical anatomy. They will see that the manual provides explanations and background information in relation to the respective practical sessions. This will allow the students to link the knowledge gained in the practical sessions to the function and clinical relevance of structures.

The contents of this course are therefore:

• Regional and Topographical Anatomy of the head and neck region, and overview of the body wall, thorax, abdomen & pelvis, upper limb and nervous system.

• Systematic Anatomy for studying the principles underlying the organisation and function of the various systems so far relevant to topographical anatomy.

• Clinical Anatomy linking topographical anatomy to clinically relevant areas.

1.2 ANATOMICAL TERMINOLOGY

Becoming aware of the anatomical position and the vocabulary used to describe various aspects of the human body is prerequisite for a studying anatomy.

• **Anatomical Position**

The anatomical position is a position used as a standard reference for describing the relation of each part of the body to each other. In the anatomical position, the patient is standing erect with the head, face and toes pointing forward, whereby the feet are together, the arms at the sides, and the palms forward (the thumb lateral).

---

*NOTE: This Manual has been **used successfully** for teaching Dental and Dental Hygiene Students from **2006-11**. The author would be grateful for **feedback** from colleagues and students for future improvements.*
email: <u>deniz.yilmazerhanke75@gmail.com</u>

1

- **Axes**

Transversal
Sagittal
Longitudinal

- **Planes**

Frontal or Coronal plane
Transverse plane or Horizontal plane
Sagittal plane - Median sagittal plane, Parasagittal plane

- **Lines**

Anteriorly:	*Posteriorly:*
Sternal line	Paravertebral line
Parasternal line	Scapular line
Medioclavicular line	Posterior axillary line
Anterior axillary line	

- **Positional terms in the whole body (trunk, limbs, head & brain)**

These terms are used in the same way in all regions of the body.

Superficial:	Towards the surface
Deep:	Towards the interior of the body or head
Ipsilateral (homolateral):	On the same side of the body or head
Contralateral:	On the opposite site of the body or head
Dexter / Dextra:	On the right
Sinister / Sinistra:	On the left
Major:	Greater
Minor:	Lesser
Superior:	Upper
Inferior:	Lower

- **Positional terms in the head including brain**

In the head and brain, the terms anterior vs. posterior and cranial vs. caudal are often used to describe the same position of a structure. Ventral structures are now localised **not** anteriorly but inferiorly, and dorsal structures superiorly.

Anterior or Cranial:	Towards the front
Posterior or Caudal:	Towards the back

Abbreviations:

ANS: autonomic nervous system; **ant.**: anterior; **CN.**: cranial nerve; **CSF**: cerebrospinal fluid; **CNS**: central nervous system; **dors.**: dorsal; **inf.**: inferior; **lat.**: lateral; **lt.**: left; **med.**: medial; **nucl.**: nucleus; **PNS**: peripheral nervous system; **post.**: posterior; **rt.**: right; **SNS**: somatic nervous system; **sup.**: superior; **TMJ**: temporomandibular joint; **ventr.**: ventral

2

- **Positional terms in the trunk and limbs**

In the body and extremities, the terms anterior versus (vs.) posterior and ventral vs. dorsal are often used synonymously to describe the position of the same structure, e.g. the anterior or ventral ramus of the spinal nerve.

Anterior or Ventral:	Towards the front of the body
Posterior or Dorsal:	Towards the back of the body
Superior or Cranial:	Towards the top of the head
Inferior or Caudal:	Towards the soles of the feet
Medial:	Closer to the midline
Lateral:	Away from the midline
Proximal or Central:	Towards the trunk
Distal or Peripheral:	Away from trunk
Palmar = Volar:	Towards the palm of the hand
Dorsal:	Away from the palm of the hand
Plantar:	Towards the sole of the foot
Dorsal:	Away from the sole of the foot
Ventral or Inferior:	Towards the feet
Dorsal or Superior:	Towards the top of the head, away from feet

- **Movements (except jaw)**

Flexion:	Anteversion bending a joint
Extension:	Retroversion straightening a joint
Abduction:	Moving away from midline
Adduction:	Moving towards midline
Medial (internal) rotation:	Anterior surface moves medially
Lateral (external) rotation:	Anterior surface moves laterally
Pronation:	Medial rotation of forearm & hand, radius crosses ulna, palm faces posteriorly
Supination:	Lateral rotation of forearm & hand, radius parallels ulna, palm faces anteriorly
Eversion:	Rotation of medial foot edge downwards, sole faces laterally
Inversion:	Rotation of medial foot edge upwards, sole faces medially
Circumduction:	Moving an extremity to form a circle

- **Movements of the jaw**

Protraction:	Move jaw anteriorly
Retraction:	Move jaw posteriorly
Elevation:	Raise superiorly
Depression:	Lower inferiorly

2. SKULL - I

We will learn the characteristics of **individual bones** forming the cranial and facial skeleton, and study the **base of the skull** superiorly and inferiorly with **structures passing through**.

2.1 PROSECTIONS AND MODELS

- **Bones of the cranial skeleton (neurocranium)**

In the cranial skeleton, we will describe the features of individual bones, their joints, and the fontanelles.

- Study the bones forming the cranial skeleton: the *frontal bone, ethmoid bone, sphenoid bone, paired parietal bones*, and *paired temporal bones* (with squamous, petrous and tympanic portions), and the *occipital bone*.
- The connection between two flat bones of the skull is a *nonsynovial fibrous joint* that is called *suture*. There are three types of sutures, the *squamous, serrated* and *denticulate sutures*. Identify the *sagittal, coronal* and *lambdoid sutures* on your skull, and name the type of these sutures.
- View a *neonatal skull* with the *fontanelles*. Find the *anterior* and *posterior fontanelle*.

The flat bones forming the *cranial vault* are also called **diploe**, because they are composed of two external layers of cortical (compact) bone, which surround the internal layer containing trabecular bone (also called cancellous or spongy bone). The cranial vault, which is formed by the flat bones of the skull, is called *exocranium*. It develops through *intramembranous ossification* (differentiation of mesenchymal tissue into bone tissue). In contrast, the cranial base, called *endocranium*, develops mainly through *endochondral ossification* (replacement of cartilaginous tissue into bone tissue). Please note that various portions of the same bone can develop in different ways, e.g. the squamous portion of the temporal bone develops through intramembranous ossification, whereas the petrous part develops through endochondral ossification.

In the *neonatal skull*, there are two frontal bones connected with the *interfrontal suture*, which ossifies later in the first year of life. The rhombic gap between the two frontal and two parietal bones covered by a membrane is called the *anterior fontanelle*, and the triangular gap between the two parietal bones and single occipital bone covered by a membrane is called the *posterior fontanelle*.

- **Bones of facial skeleton (viscerocranium)**

- Describe characteristics of the **paired bones**, which are the *maxillae, zygomatic bones, lacrimal bone, nasal bones, palatine bones*, and the *inferior conchae*.

- View the *mandible, vomer,* and *hyoid bone*, which occur as **single bones** in the **adult**.
- Identify the **portions** of the *frontal, ethmoid* and *sphenoid bones* **contributing to the facial skeleton**.

The facial skeleton lies anterior to the cranial base, and shapes **three cavities**: the *orbit, nasal cavity* and *oral cavity*. Whereas the first two cavities are embedded in the skull bone, the oral cavity is formed by the skull and mandible, which are connected through a joint and soft tissue (cheeks, floor of the mouth). In addition, the *pterygopalatine* and *infratemporal fossae* are interposed between the cranial and facial skeletons.

Some parts of the facial skeleton develop through *intramembranous ossification*, others through *endochondral ossification*. One very special type of bone development in the facial skeleton involves the development of a bone through *intramembranous ossification along a cartilaginous track*, e.g. the mandible develops through intramembranous ossification along the Meckel's cartilage.

- **Base of skull (superior view) and structures passing through**

We will first view the *anterior, middle* and *posterior* **cranial fossae** on the superior aspect of the skull base. In a next step, we will identify the **cranial nerves, arteries and veins passing through foramina, canals, fissures, etc.** of the skull base. There are *twelve cranial nerves*, which are numbered from *CN. I* to *CN. XII*.

- The *brainstem* leaves the intracranial cavity through the **foramen magnum**. Its continuation, the *spinal cord*, courses in the vertebral canal.
- **CN. I**: Inspect the crista galli of the ethmoid bone and the **cribriform plate**, through which the *olfactory nerve fibres (CN. I)* pass on their way from the nasal cavity to the anterior cranial fossa. The *anterior meningeal artery*, however, leaves the anterior cranial fossa towards the nasal cavity by coursing in the opposite direction, where it supplies the nasal mucosa. The anterior meningeal artery is a branch of the anterior ethmoidal artery, which we will learn in more detail, when we study the orbit.
- **CN. II**: The *optic nerve (CN. II)* passes through the **optic canal** together with the *ophthalmic artery*.
- **CN. III, IV, V_1, and VI**: The **superior orbital fissure** connects the middle cranial fossa with the orbit. The *oculomotor nerve (CN. III), trochlear nerve (CN. IV)* and *abducens nerve (CN. VI)* supplying the skeletal muscles of the eye as well as the sensory *ophthalmic nerve (CN. V_1)*, which is the first branch of the trigeminal nerve (CN. V), run through this fissure together with the *superior ophthalmic vein*.
- **CN. V_2**: The second branch of the trigeminal nerve called the *maxillary nerve (CN. V_2)* leaves the intracranial cavity through the **foramen rotundum**.
- **CN. V_3**: The third branch of the trigeminal nerve called the *mandibular nerve (CN. V_3)* leaves the intracranial cavity through the **foramen ovale**.

- Just lateral to the foramen ovale, there is a small hole called **foramen spinosum**, through which the *middle meningeal artery* (branch of maxillary artery) enters the intracranial cavity, and courses together with the *meningeal branch of the mandibular nerve*. Starting at the foramen spinosum trace the grooves of the branches of the middle meningeal artery, the thickest periostal artery in the cranial vault. View also the *pterion* in the region of the *sphenoid fontanelle*, which intersects the course of the anterior division of the middle meningeal artery. It is localised at the junction of the greater wing of the sphenoid, squamous temporal, frontal, and parietal bones.
- **CN. VII and VIII:** Two cranial nerves, the *facial nerve (CN. VII)* and *vestibulocochlear nerve (CN. VIII)*, enter the **internal acoustic meatus** together with the *labyrinthine vessels*. Whereas the vestibulocochlear nerve heads towards the inner ear (bony and membranous labyrinth) the facial nerve has a more complicated course.

  The facial nerve has a small trunk called **nervus intermedius** with sensory (gustatory) and autonomic components. One *autonomic branch* of the nervus intermedius is the *greater petrosal nerve*, which leaves the facial nerve at the *geniculate ganglion* embedded in the petrosal part of the temporal bone, and passes through its own hiatus (**hiatus of the greater petrosal nerve**) to re-enter the intracranial cavity.

  A *second branch* of the nervus intermedius (from CN. VII) is the *chorda tympani nerve*, which has *gustatory and autonomic components*. It leaves the facial nerve in the air-filled cavity of the middle ear (tympanic cavity), and therefore it is called chorda tympani nerve, meaning the thread (=chord) of the tympanic cavity. It courses anteriorly between two interconnected small bones (ossicles) called malleus and incus. Finally, it leaves the skull through the **petrotympanic fissure** (*Glaser*) at the inferior aspect of the skull base. The *last (motor) portion* of the *facial nerve* passes through the **stylomastoid foramen**, which can be seen on the inferior aspect of the skull base.
- Please note that the inner opening of the **carotid canal** is just lateral to the **foramen lacerum**. The *internal carotid artery* courses directly above the foramen lacerum after it enters the intracranial cavity through the carotid canal together with the *internal carotid nerve plexus*, the latter coursing in the wall of the artery (postganglionic sympathetic fibres in the tunica adventitia, see **Histology** books). The size and form of the foramen lacerum is subject to high interindividual variation, and in the living patient it is filled with fibrocartilage.

  Since the foramen lacerum is in the immediate vicinity of the carotid canal, sympathetic nerve fibres leaving the internal carotid plexus in the carotid canal can **join** the greater petrosal nerve after it enters the foramen lacerum. These postganglionic sympathetic nerve fibres are called the *deep petrosal nerve*. The nerve resulting from the fusion of the greater petrosal <u>and</u> deep petrosal nerves exits the intracranial cavity as the *Vidian nerve of the pterygoid canal* by entering the **pterygoid canal** through the foramen lacerum. From here, the Vidian nerve heads towards the pterygopalatine fossa (see next session).

CN. IX: The *lesser petrosal nerve* leaves the middle cranial fossa through the foramen lacerum, and from here it exits the intracranial cavity to reach the otic ganglion. The lesser petrosal nerve is the end branch of the *tympanic nerve (Jacobson)* from the *glossopharyngeal nerve (CN. IX)*. It re-enters the petrous part of the temporal bone through the **tympanic canaliculus** after the glossopharyngeal nerve has left the skull through the jugular foramen (see below). The tympanic canaliculus has its opening in the *petrous fossula*, which can be seen at the inferior aspect of the skull base between the outer openings of the carotid canal and the jugular foramen.

- **CN. IX, X and XI:** Altogether three cranial nerves, the *glossopharyngeal nerve (CN. IX)*, *vagus nerve (CN. X)* and *accessory nerve (CN. XI)* exit the posterior cranial fossa through the **anterior part** of the **jugular foramen**, whereas the internal jugular vein passes through the **posterior part** of the jugular foramen (jugular bulb).
- **CN. XII:** The hypoglossal nerve (CN. XII) passes through the **hypoglossal canal**.

The **branchial arches (pharyngeal arches)** are the **anlage** for *skeletal, muscular* and *connective tissue* elements in the skull and neck that are supplied by the *respective branchial nerves* and *blood vessels*. Therefore, the motor supply to these muscles is also called *"branchial motor"* innervation.

Structures that develop from the **1st branchial arch** are all innervated by the *maxillary* and *mandibular nerves* [maxilla, Meckel's cartilage (for the aiding development of mandible), ossicles in the middle ear (malleus, incus), the sphenomandibular ligament, and muscles supplied by the mandibular nerve (tensor tympani & tensor veli palatini, muscles of mastication, mylohyoid & anterior belly of digastric)]. The **2nd branchial arch** gives rise to the Reichert's cartilage (for the stapes in the middle ear, styloid process, stylohyoid ligament & lesser horn of hyoid bone), and muscles supplied by the *motor division of the facial nerve* (stapedius, stylohyoid, posterior belly of the digastric, muscles of facial expression incl. buccinator & platysma). The *glossopharyngeal nerve* is the nerve of the **3rd branchial arch**, from which the stylopharyngeus muscle and greater horn of the hyoid bone and lower part its body develop. The **4th branchial arch** provides material for the development of laryngeal cartilages (thyroid cartilage & epiglottis), the cricothyroid muscle, and intrinsic muscles of soft palate (all except tensor veli palatini innervated by the mandibular nerve), all supplied by the *superior laryngeal branch of the vagus nerve*. Structures that develop from the **6th branchial arch** are the remaining laryngeal cartilages (cricoid, arytenoid & corniculate cartilages) and muscles (except cricothyroid muscle) innervated by the *recurrent laryngeal branch of the vagus nerve*.

NOTE: You should carefully study the skull base and learn the course of the nerves and vessels. The course of autonomic branches innervating the salivary glands will be reconstructed in the last practical session of the head and neck region.

- **Base of skull (inferior view) and structures passing through**

Identify the foramina, canals, etc. studied above on the inferior aspect of the skull. These will be the *foramen ovale, foramen spinosum, foramen lacerum, carotid canal, jugular foramen*, and *hypoglossal canal*. Some foramina, however, will have their exits in other areas, e.g. the foramen rotundum & pterygoid canal lead to the pterygopalatine fossa. Now you can view the following structures on the inferior skull base:

- Inspect the bones of the **hard palate** with the *transverse palatine suture* between the *palatine* and *maxillary bones*. The *median palatine suture* is localised between the right (rt.) and left (lt.) maxillae, and separates also the rt. and lt. palatine bones. Find the *incisive foramen*, and the *greater and lesser palatine foramina*.
- Identify the *choanes* and the *vomer*.
- Find the *med. and lat. plates* of the **pterygoid process** with the *pterygoid fossa* between them, and the *pterygoid hamulus* emerging from the medial plate of the pterygoid process in the sphenoid bone.
- See the **styloid process, mastoid process,** and **stylomastoid foramen** in the temporal bone.
- View the **petrotympanic fissure** (*Glaser*) and, if it can be seen, also the *petrosquamous fissure* between the different parts of the temporal bone (between the petrous and tympanic parts, and between the petrous and squamous parts, respectively). If both fissures can be seen, the petrotympanic fissure will lie more posteriorly than the petrosquamous fissure.
- View the groove for the **pharyngotympanic (auditory or Eustachian) tube**.
- Find the external openings of the *carotid canal* and the *jugular foramen* at the *jugular fossa*. The *petrous fossula* with the **tympanic canaliculus** lies between the two openings. The **apertura externa aquaeductus cochleae** lies just behind the petrous fossula.
- View the **mastoid canaliculus**, where the *auricular branch* of the *vagus nerve* (CN. X) re-enters the skull.

During development the *main parts of the two maxillae* are connected with the *incisive bone* (originating from the primary palate) via the *incisive suture*, the latter suture also found in some adult skulls. The incisive suture runs *from the incisive canal* to the anterior surface of the maxilla, where it courses *between the lateral incisor and the canine tooth* (synonyms of incisive bone: intermaxillary bone, premaxillary bone).

Primary or anterior palate clefts (described as a "cleft lip" or "hare lip") occur when the incisive bone develops incompletely. *Secondary or posterior palate clefts* occur when the two lateral palatine processes of the maxilla fail to fuse in the midline and/or with the nasal septum, where the three structures meet each other. If the anterior and posterior palate clefts concur, this leads to the most severe malformations of the palate.

3. SKULL - II

In the second skull session, we will study **skulls with** (mainly dura mater) **and without meninges**. The practical session will focus on the *meninges and venous sinuses*, and the *bones of the facial skeleton*. In the facial skeleton, we will inspect bones forming and/or surrounding the *orbit, nasal cavity, paranasal air sinuses, infratemporal fossa* and *pterygopalatine fossa*.

3.1 PROSECTIONS AND MODELS

- **Meninges (and their contribution to formation of venous sinuses)**

The meninges of the brain consist of three membranes separating the epidural, subdural and subarachnoid spaces from each other.

- View the innermost **pia mater**, which is a thin membrane adhering to the surface of the brain and follows the contours of the gyri and sulci.
- Examine the outermost **dura mater**, which is a thick, dense and tough membrane adhering to the inner portion of bones forming the intracranial cavity. It consists of an external *periostal* (parietal) and internal *meningeal* (visceral) layer, which are attached to each other. However, the two layers separate to form **venous sinuses**. In addition the *falx cerebri, tentorium cerebelli* and *falx cerebelli* are dural extensions formed by attachments of two meningeal (visceral) layers of dura mater. It should also be noted that the dura mater is the *periosteum* of the inner portion of *cranial bones*, which becomes detached from the bones in the adult skull except at the sutures.
- Inspect the **arachnoid membrane**, which courses directly below the dura mater, but does not adhere to it. It sends out *arachnoid trabeculae* (columns of connective tissue) adhering to the pia mater. Near the *vertex of the brain*, the arachnoid membrane penetrates the meningeal layer of the dura mater, and sends off extensions into the venous sinuses called *arachnoid granulations*. These flower-shaped granulations drain the *cerebrospinal fluid* from the subarachnoid space (see below) back into the venous system. Therefore, the cerebrospinal fluid is also regarded as the *lymph of the brain*.

- **Spaces between the meninges and skull bone**

- Identify the space between the cranial bones and dura mater corresponding to the **epidural space**.
- Inspect the space between the dura mater and arachnoid membrane. This space is a very thin capillary gap called the **subdural space**.
- View the space between the arachnoid membrane and pia mater called the **subarachnoid space.** It extends from below the arachnoid membrane to the pia mater, whereby it reaches the surface of the brain including the gyri and depths of the sulci.

Periostal arteries of the cranial vault (e.g. the middle meningeal artery) course in the epidural space. Their rupture, e.g. following a fracture of the cranial skeleton can cause an *epidural haemorrhage* (arterial bleeding).

Diploic veins, which reside in the internal layer of the diploe between the two external (cortical) layers, drain through *emissary veins* either into intracranial venous sinuses or extracranial veins of the head. If the external compact layer of the diploe is completely removed, the four major diploic veins running in the internal layer of the diploe can be seen (frontal, anterior temporal, posterior temporal and occipital diploic veins).

Superior cerebral veins draining the brain also discharge into the venous sinuses. Because they course in the subarachnoid space they have to penetrate first the arachnoid membrane, then pass the subdural space, and finally penetrate the meningeal layer of the dura mater before they can enter/join a venous sinus. These (soft) veins can easily be torn during their passage through the (hard) meningeal layer of the dura mater, and rupture in case of a traumatic event leading to a *subdural haematoma* (venous bleeding).

Enlargements of the subarachnoid space are called *cisterns* (e.g. cerebellomedullary cistern). The subarachnoid space is filled with *cerebrospinal fluid* and also contains *blood vessels* coursing on the brain surface before they enter the nervous tissue they supply. Therefore, the cerebrospinal fluid will contain blood following rupture of cerebral vessels coursing in the subarachnoid space. This event called *subarachnoid haemorrhage* is usually an arterial bleeding caused by a rupture of an aneurysm (sac of arterial wall).

- **Major venous sinuses, sella turcica and pituitary fossa**

- Identify the grooves of the *superior sagittal, transverse, sigmoid* and *occipital* sinuses on a skull without meninges.

- Now take the skull containing the dura mater and view the *superior sagittal sinus* and *arachnoid granulations* at the insertion of the falx cerebri. The *inferior sagittal sinus* runs at the inferior margin of the falx cerebri, and drains into the *confluence of sinuses* via the *straight sinus*.

- In the sphenoid bone, identify the *sella turcica* with its anterior and posterior *margins*, and the *ant. & post. clinoid processes* on a skull without meninges. Between the anterior and posterior margins of the sella turcica you will see the *pituitary fossa*, which contains a gland called the *pituitary gland (hypophysis)*. The pituitary gland is covered superiorly by a *diaphragm* formed by the dura mater. The posterior margin of the sella turcica is also the beginning of the *clivus* formed by the sphenoid and occipital bones, on which the brainstem resides.

- The *cavernous sinus* is an irregular network of small venous sinuses, which lies around the pituitary gland. The rt. and lt. cavernous sinuses are connected with each other.

- The oculomotor (CN. III), trochlear (CN. IV), and abducens nerves (CN. VI), and the sensory ophthalmic nerve (CN. V_1), which course towards the superior orbital fissure on their way to the orbit, as well as the maxillary nerve (CN. V_2) all have a section that is *embedded* in the **cavernous sinus**. In addition, the internal carotid artery *passes directly through* the cavernous sinus.

- The *superior petrosal sinus* drains/connects the cavernous sinus (in)to the transverse and sigmoid sinuses, and the *inferior petrosal sinus* into the internal jugular vein.

Damage to the nerves supplying the orbit during their common course through the cavernous sinus can lead to a **complete ophthalmoplegia** (paralysis or weakness of all muscles that control eye movement as well as the eye sensation including loss of the corneal reflex).

- **Foramina, canals and fissures for emissary veins**

Remember that **emissary veins** pass *through the skull bone*, and *connect* the intracranial and extracranial venous systems.

- *Mastoid foramen* (emissary vein connecting sigmoid sinus with occipital vein),
- *Occipital foramen* (emissary vein connecting confluence of sinuses at the external occipital protuberance with occipital vein),
- *Parietal foramen* (emissary vein connecting superior sagittal sinus with a parietal branch of the superficial temporal vein),
- *Condylar canal* (emissary vein connecting sigmoid sinus with the external vertebral venous plexus in the vicinity of the jugular foramen),
- *Superior orbital fissure* (superior ophthalmic vein connecting cavernous sinus with several facial veins, e.g. angular vein),
- *Foramen ovale* and *carotid canal* (venous plexuses connecting cavernous sinus with pterygoid plexus),
- *Hypoglossal canal* (emissary vein connecting *basilar* and *marginal venous plexuses* with the internal jugular vein.

Emissary veins drain the blood into both intracranial and extracranial directions depending on the actual intracranial and outer pressure, because intracranial venous sinuses do not have valves. Therefore, they can pave the way for spreading of infections from extracranial regions to intracranial venous sinuses. For example, a *cavernous sinus thrombosis* can result from **infections carried into the cavernous sinus** from the face, **teeth**, palatine region, paranasal air sinuses or pharyngeal region through the *superior ophthalmic vein* or *pterygoid plexus*.

- **Bones of the orbit**

The orbit contains the *eye ball, eye muscles, lacrimal gland,* and *ciliary ganglion* as well as *nerves and vessels*. It is connected with regions located in both the cranial and facial skeleton.

- Inspect the **boundaries of the orbit**: The **roof** of the orbit is formed by the *frontal bone*, and its **lateral margin** by the *zygomatic bone*. Together with the *maxilla*, the zygomatic bone also forms the **floor** of the orbit. The *frontal process of the maxilla* contributes to the **medial border** of the orbit. The **posterior wall** of the orbit is formed by the *lesser and greater wings* of the *sphenoid bone* as well as by the *ethmoid* and *lacrimal bones*, the *maxilla* and sometimes a tiny *orbital process of the palatine bone*.
- View the *supraorbital* and *supratrochlear foramina* (or notches) and the *zygomaticoorbital foramen* (also zygomatic canal).
- Inspect the *superior orbital fissure* formed by the *lesser and greater wings* of the *sphenoid bone,* and the *optic canal* connecting the orbit with the intracranial cavity.
- The *inferior orbital fissure* connecting the orbit with the pterygopalatine fossa is localised between the greater wing of the sphenoid bone, zygomatic bone, and maxilla.
- The *infraorbital groove* is the proximal portion of the *infraorbital canal*, which has its exit at the *infraorbital foramen*.

• **Nasal cavity and paranasal air sinuses**

- Inspect the **connections of the nasal cavity** to the anterior cranial fossa through the *cribriform plate* of the ethmoid bone and to the nasopharynx through the *choanae*. Blood vessels from the pterygopalatine fossa reach the nasal cavity through the *sphenopalatine foramen*. The *nasolacrimal duct* drains tears from the orbit to nasal cavity (inferior nasal meatus).
- View the **boundaries of the nasal cavity**: The **roof** (cribriform plate of the ethmoid bone, nasal spine of the frontal bone, nasal bones and cartilages), **floor** (palatal processes of maxilla and palatine bone), **lateral wall** (sup. and middle conchae formed by the ethmoid bone, other parts of the ethmoid bone, inf. nasal concha, palatine bone, maxilla and sphenoid bone), and the **nasal septum in the middle** (septal cartilages, vertical plate of ethmoid bone, vomer).
- View the *superior, middle and inferior meatus* localised below the respective conchae, and the *sphenoethmoid recess* above the superior nasal concha.
- Find the **openings of the paranasal air sinuses** at the lateral wall of the nasal cavity: openings of posterior ethmoidal air cells in the *superior meatus*, of the sphenoid sinus at the *sphenoethmoid recess*, and of the frontal sinus, maxillary sinus and anterior ethmoidal air cells at the *hiatus semilunaris* extending below the *bulla ethmoidalis*.

Fractures of the *cribriform plate* (frontal bone) can cause *liquorrhea* (cerebrospinal fluid dropping out of the nose), when the *dura & arachnoid membrane* are damaged. This condition is a serious risk for *meningitis* and has to be treated surgically.

Pituitary gland tumours restricted to the *sella turcica* can be surgically approached through the *nasal cavity* and *sphenoid sinus*.

In addition, infections in the sphenoid air sinus (see below) can directly penetrate the cavernous sinus through the posterior wall of the sphenoidal sinus leading to a *cavernous sinus thrombosis*. Likewise, a *sigmoid sinus thrombosis* may result from infections of the middle ear cavity (infiltration from mastoid cells connected to the middle air cavity).

- **Infratemporal and pterygopalatine fossae**

The **pterygopalatine fossa** is a narrow cleft localised between the posterior wall of the maxilla and the pterygoid process of the sphenoid bone. It has a very **strategic position**, because it connects many important areas.

- View the **connections** of the pterygopalatine fossa

a) to the *middle cranial fossa*. The maxillary nerve coming through the *foramen rotundum* and the nerve of the pterygoid canal (Vidian) coming through the *pterygoid canal* meet in the pterygopalatine fossa to join at the pterygopalatine ganglion. The *entrance* of the pterygoid canal itself lies within the *foramen lacerum*, where the greater petrosal nerve leaves the middle cranial fossa towards the pterygopalatine ganglion, and joins postganglionic sympathetic fibres (deep petrosal nerve) to form the Vidian nerve in the pterygoid canal.

b) to the *orbit* through the *inferior orbital fissure* (for the infraorbital nerve from the maxillary nerve and the inferior ophthalmic vein),

c) to the *nasal cavity* through the *sphenopalatine foramen* (for the sphenopalatine artery, which is the end branch of the maxillary artery),

d) to the *hard palate* through the *greater and lesser palatine canals* (for the nerves and vessels), and *incisive foramen* (for the nasopalatine nerve),

e) and to *infratemporal fossa* through the *pterygomaxillary fissure*, which is the lateral opening of the pterygopalatine fossa.

- Identity the **borders of the infratemporal fossa**:

(a) The **roof** of the infratemporal fossa is formed by the horizontal portion of the greater wing of the sphenoid bone.

(b) Find the **remaining borders** of the infratemporal fossa. It extends from the posterior surface of the maxilla (**anterior border**) to the foramen ovale and foramen spinosum **posteriorly**. Its **lateral wall** is formed by the mandibular ramus. **Medially** it extends to the lateral pterygoid plate, and maxilla, where it is also connected through the *pterygomaxillary fissure* with the pterygopalatine fossa. Thus, structures coming from the pterygopalatine fossa can reach the infratemporal fossa and vice versa (e.g. sphenopalatine artery).

NOTE: The infratemporal fossa contains the *maxillary artery, venous pterygoid plexus, proximal portion of the mandibular nerve* giving rise to its divisions (where they branch further) & *two muscles of mastication with their nerves and blood vessels* (med. & lat. pterygoids). These structures will be studied later.

4. MUSCLES OF FACIAL EXPRESSION

The aim is to **remove the skin** for dissecting the *muscles of facial expression* and the course of the *facial nerve* **on the face**. We will also dissect the *cervical branch* (ramus colli) of the facial nerve by removing the skin of the **neck anteriorly**.

4.1 DISSECTIONS

- **Removal of the skin**

- First remove the skin of the head and neck anteriorly. By doing so, note differences in the thickness of the skin at different locations, and inspect the subcutaneous tissue below the skin.

- In the face and anterior neck you will encounter the muscles of facial expression below the skin.

> The muscles of facial expression are skin muscles (the only skin muscles in humans) defined by their origin at bones and their insertion in the skin. During removal of the skin in the face take care of these muscles, and branches of the facial nerve, which innervate them (motor nerve). Use an anatomical atlas to identify the muscles and to avoid their accidental removal.

- **Muscles of facial expression and facial nerve**

- **In the face**, dissect the *temporal, zygomatic, buccal, marginal mandibular* and *cervical* **branches of the facial nerve** (CN.VII) while you **remove the fascia** of the *muscles of facial expression*.

- Identify the occipitofrontalis (epicranius), ant. auricular, orbicularis oculi, corrugator supercilii, procerus and levator labii sup. alaeque nasi muscles (the post. and sup. auricular muscles are attached to the skin at back of the head).

- Study carefully the muscles involved in *chewing and other movements of the mouth*. They are the buccinator, zygomaticus major and minor, risorius, orbicularis oris, levator labii superioris, levator anguli oris, depressor labii inferioris, depressor anguli oris, and mentalis muscles.

- **In the neck**, dissect the *platysma*, which draws the skin of the neck up, and can also pull the lower lip and corners of the mouth downwards.

- **Blood vessels of the face and auriculotemporal nerve**

- Dissect the **facial artery**, which has a tortuous course at the chin, with all of its branches including the *angular artery*.

- Dissect the **superficial temporal artery and vein** as well as the thin **auriculotemporal nerve**, which courses together with the vessels, although the vessels are located more posteriorly. Find and palpate the superficial temporal artery **on your own temple**.

- Dissect the following **branches** of the superficial temporal artery: *transverse facial artery*, as well as *frontal, middle temporal* and *parietal branches*. The smaller (but not less important) branches supplying the temporomandibular joint (TMJ, via *articular branches*), zygomatic arch and orbit (via *zygomatico-orbital branches*) are more difficult to preserve.

- **Delineate the areas**, which receive a sensory innervation from the auriculotemporal nerve (temporomandibular joint, auricle, external auditory meatus, and skin of the temple and lateral scalp).

Frey's syndrome (also known as auriculotemporal syndrome or gustatory sweating) is characterised by hyperesthesia, flushing and warmth or sweating in the skin area supplied by the auriculotemporal nerve and/or greater auricular nerve. The triggering stimulus is eating foods, which induce a strong salivation. The cause is usually a lesion of the TMJ or a condylar fracture of the mandible.

- **Superficial blood vessels and nerves in the anterior neck region**

- **Before you continue dissection, search for** the external jugular vein on your class mate's / colleague's neck with the aid of surface markings (e.g. mandible and the anterior border of the sternocleidomastoid muscle).

- Dissect the **external jugular vein** along its oblique course on the sternocleidomastoid muscle from the lobe of the ear to the posterior cervical triangle. **Do not damage the *transverse cervical vein***, which usually drains into the external jugular vein (alternatively, it can also drain directly into the subclavian vein).

The external jugular vein is important to assess cardiac function, as it runs superficially. In right heart failure, it is congested already at a 45°angle of the body and neck.

- Now find the so-called **nerve point** (*punctum nervosum*) by lifting the *platysma* distally. The *nerve point* is located approximately at the midpoint of the *posterolateral border* of the *sternocleidomastoid muscle*. It marks the general region where the *cutaneous branches of the cervical plexus* emerge into the subcutaneous tissues of the neck, i.e. the lesser occipital, greater auricular, transverse cervical, and supraclavicular nerves (**see Anterior Neck Practical Session**).

- In this session, we will only clean up the **transverse cervical nerve**, which courses with the *transverse cervical artery and vein*. Thus, you can find the transverse cervical nerve easily by tracing the transverse cervical vein back to the external jugular vein.

- Search for the *anastomosis* of the *cervical branch of the facial nerve* with the *transverse cervical nerve*, which form the **superficial cervical ansa** for the *motor innervation* of the *platysma* (from cervical branch of the facial nerve), and *sensory innervation* of the *platysma and skin of the neck* (from transverse cervical nerve).

4.2 PROSECTIONS AND MODELS

• **Facial nerve**

- Identify the temporal, zygomatic, buccal, marginal mandibular and cervical *branches of the facial nerve (CN.VII)* and locate the *duct of the parotid gland*.

- Identify the *muscles of facial expression* as described above. The muscles of facial expression receive a **motor innervation from the facial nerve (CN. VII)**.

- Search for the *origin* of the muscles on the *facial skeleton*.

- Learn about the function of muscles of facial expression by **imitating the movements** yourself.

- View the *posterior belly of the digastric muscle* and the *stylohyoid muscle* innervated by the *facial nerve*. In addition to these muscles, the facial nerve also innervates the *stapedius muscle* in the middle ear.

5. FACIAL PLEXUS, ORAL CAVITY, TEETH AND SALIVARY GLANDS

Today, we will **dissect the trunk of the facial nerve** by tracing the *peripheral branches* of the facial nerve back. We will demonstrate that the trunk of the facial nerve leaves the skull at the *stylomastoid foramen*. We will also identify some sensory **branches of the trigeminal nerve supplying the skin.**

In addition, we will **remove the zygomatic arch** in order to open the temporomandibular joint and approach the infratemporal fossa in the next practical session. A major part of this session, however, focuses on the **living and topographical anatomy** of the *oral cavity, teeth,* and *salivary glands* to be studied in **prosections.**

5.1 DISSECTIONS

- **End branches of trigeminal nerve**

- Dissect the **main end branches** of the **three divisions of the trigeminal nerve:** the *supraorbital* and *supratrochlear nerves* from the ophthalmic nerve (CN. V_1), the *infraorbital* nerve from the maxillary nerve (CN. V_2), and the *mental nerve* from the mandibular nerve (CN. V_3).

> The mental nerve is the continuation of the inferior alveolar nerve, which innervates the teeth of the mandibular arch. Therefore, during surgery on the lower teeth the skin of the *chin and lower lip* supplied by the mental nerve becomes *numb* after *anaesthesia of the inferior alveolar nerve.*

- **Plexus of facial nerve within parotid gland**

- Remove the *buccal sucking fat pad* and mobilise the **duct of the parotid gland** by avoiding damage the duct (If you see branches of the buccal nerve, preserve them).

- Follow the *distal branches* of the facial nerve **up to the point where they leave the parotid gland** (temporal, zygomatic, buccal, marginal mandibular and cervical branches of the facial nerve).

- **Cut out** a large **U-shaped piece of parotid tissue around the duct**, and **reflect the duct** medially with **the glandular tissue.**

- Now, you can **remove** the remnants of the **superficial portion of the parotid gland** by cutting them radially. Hereby, **try to preserve** as many as of the branches of the facial nerve (CN.VII) and **expose** the **plexus of the facial nerve** within the gland. You will see that the plexus spreads out in a single plane, which is interposed between the superficial and deep portions of the parotid gland.

17

- **Trunk of the facial nerve and retromandibular vein**

- Proceed to this step, after you have dissected the plexus of the facial nerve within the parotid gland, and have reflected the parotid duct with parotid tissue medially.

- Now, we will follow the facial nerve until the point, where it leaves the skull at the **stylomastoid foramen**. Remove the remnants of the parotid gland, and clean the tissue above the masseter muscle.

- Also dissect the **retromandibular vein** and the **facial vein**.

With the aid of the plexus, the facial nerve **distributes** autonomic and sensory nerve fibres within the parotid gland. The *autonomic fibres* (**secretory fibres**) coursing with the facial nerve do not originate from the facial nerve but from the *glossopharyngeal nerve (lesser petrosal branch)*, and are carried from the *otic ganglion* to the parotid gland by the *auriculotemporal nerve* (branch of CN. V_3). The *sensory innervation* to the **connective tissue** of the parotid gland originates directly from the *auriculotemporal nerve,* and to the **parotid capsule** from the *auriculotemporal & great auricular nerves (anatomical variation)*. The facial nerve itself provides the motor innervation to the muscles of facial expression.

A **parotid gland tumour** can therefore cause a *peripheral facial nerve palsy* and disturbances in the *autonomic innervation* in some or all parts of the gland depending on its location. As a result, only those muscles of facial expression will be paralysed, which are innervated by the branches affected.

A **lesion of the facial nerve before it receives autonomic fibres** from the auriculotemporal nerve (e.g. before the facial nerve leaves the stylomastoid foramen) will therefore not necessarily affect the autonomic innervation of the parotid gland (if the distal portions of facial nerve do not degenerate). A *Bell's palsy* (sudden **peripheral facial nerve palsy**) may result from a degenerative or inflammatory injury to the facial nerve after it exits the brainstem. The palsy is always *ipsilateral* to the lesion and usually affects the whole facial nerve including the branches supplying the frontal and orbicularis oculi muscles. These branches are preserved in *supranuclear facial nerve palsy*, where the lower branches of the facial nerve are paralysed *contralateral* to the central lesion (lesion in the central nervous system). The **parotid region** includes the *parotid gland*, the *facial nerve, maxillary artery, retromandibular vein, auriculotemporal nerve*, and *superficial temporal artery*. The **parotid gland itself** is covered by a *capsule* (or *fascia*, extremely painful in parotitis, e.g. in mumps) and lies superficial to the masseter muscle. From there it extends posteriorly into the retromandibular fossa (delineated by the ramus of the mandible, sternocleidomastoid muscle and external acoustic meatus) up to the styloid process, superiorly to the zygomatic process, and inferiorly to the angle of the mandible. **Local anaesthesia** of the *inferior alveolar nerve* can extend up to the parotid region affecting its contents, and thereby causing temporary or permanent **facial nerve palsy**.

- • **Removal of zygomatic arch**
- **Remove the fascia** of the *masseter* and *temporal muscles*.
- At the origin of the two heads of the masseter muscle (along the zygomatic arch) **search for the masseteric nerve** (a very thin nerve) embedded in the superficial portion of the tendon.
- Dissect the masseter muscle and nerve from the zygomatic arch.
- **Remove about 3-4 cm** of the *zygomatic arch* by sawing it. Start at the articular eminence next to the TMJ.
- Now, displace the masseter muscle from the ramus of the mandible up to the angle, but do not remove the muscle from the mandibular bone. The masseter muscle should be **kept attached to the angle of the mandible**, and finally **reflected caudally** (downwards).

5.2 PROSECTIONS AND MODELS

- • **Oral cavity**
- **Look in each others' mouth**. Identify the *frenulum* of the *tongue*, the *frenulum* of the *lips*, the *vestibules*, the *sublingual folds* and the *deep lingual vein*. View also **openings of the salivary glands**: the *parotid papilla* with the *opening of the parotid duct* (opposite to 2nd maxillary molar), the *sublingual caruncle* with the *opening of the submandibular duct*, and the *sublingual fold* with *openings of the sublingual glands* (on the inferior surface and apex of the tongue).
- Examine the **roof of the mouth**. As the person says 'ah' note the elevation of the **soft palate**. Identify the *oropharyngeal isthmus*, the *palatoglossal and palatopharyngeal arches*, the *palatine tonsils*, and the *uvula*.

Summary of the sensory innervation of the oral cavity

Hard and soft palate: The *nasopalatine (long sphenopalatine) nerve* supplies the lingual gingiva and palatal mucosa anterior to the maxillary canines and the *greater palatine nerve* posterior to the maxillary canines. The *lesser palatine nerve* supplies the soft palate.

Upper vestibular (labial/buccal) gingiva: The *anterior superior alveolar nerve* supplies the vestibular gingiva of the maxillary incisors and canines, the *middle superior alveolar nerve* of the maxillary premolars, and the *posterior superior alveolar nerve* of the maxillary molars.

Mucosa of the cheek: *Buccal nerve.*

Lower vestibular (labial/buccal) gingiva: The *mental nerve* (end branch of inferior alveolar nerve) supplies the vestibular gingiva of the mandibular incisors, and the *buccal nerve* the vestibular gingiva of the molar region.

Floor of the mouth and lower lingual gingiva: The *lingual nerve* supplies the lingual gingiva of the mandibular teeth.

- **Hard and soft palate**

- View the *palatoglossal* and *palatopharyngeal muscles* forming the palatoglossal and palatopharyngeal arches, and the *levator veli palatini, tensor veli palatini* and *uvular muscles.*

- **All palatine muscles except the tensor veli palatini muscle** receive their motor innervation from the *cranial portion* of the *accessory nerve (CN. XI)*, which reach the palatine (and pharyngeal) muscles via the vagus nerve (CN. X), after the cranial portion of the accessory nerve has joined the vagus nerve in the jugular foramen *(communicating branch of accessory nerve)*. The *tensor veli palatini muscle* is supplied by the *mandibular nerve (CN. V$_3$)*.

- View the *ascending palatine artery* and *facial artery*, which **supply the palatine tonsils**. Also find the *ascending pharyngeal, lesser palatine* and *dorsal lingual arteries* contributing to the blood supply of the palatine tonsils. Study the *lymphatic drainage* of palatine tonsils (retropharyngeal and deep parotid lymph nodes).

The *lingual tonsil, pharyngeal tonsil* (adenoids), *paired lateral bands* (along the salpingopharyngeal folds), *paired tubal tonsils* (at the pharyngeal opening of the Eustachian tube), and the *paired palatine tonsils* form a **ring of lymphatic tissue** (lymphatic tissue of Waldeyer's tonsillar ring) between the nasopharynx and oropharynx.

- **Dentition**

- View the **structure** of upper and lower teeth (permanent and deciduous) in the respective dental arches.

- **Number** the teeth according to various forms of Dental charting.

- View dental **anomalies** (e.g. supernumerary teeth, microdontia, periodontitis).

- Inspect the innervation of the **upper (maxillary) teeth** by the:

   1) *anterior superior alveolar nerves* (maxillary incisors and canines),

   2) *middle superior alveolar nerves* (maxillary premolars and the mesiobuccal root of the 1st maxillary molar),

   3) and the *posterior superior alveolar nerves* (maxillary molars except the mesiobuccal root of the 1st maxillary molar)

- Inspect the innervation of the **lower (mandibular) teeth** by the *inferior alveolar nerve* (including the incisive branch from the mental nerve to the lateral and central incisors).

Dental occlusion describes the manner, in which the teeth in the upper (maxillary) and lower (mandibular) jaws contact each other in the mouth closed.

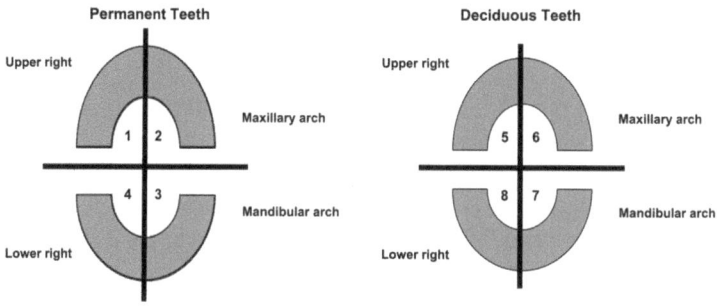

Permanent Teeth

right upper	**18 17 16** <u>15</u> <u>14</u> **13** *12 11*	*21 22 23* <u>24</u> <u>25</u> **26 27 28**	left upper
right lower	**48 47 46** <u>45</u> <u>44</u> **43** *42 41*	*31 32 33* <u>34</u> <u>35</u> **36 37 38**	left lower

Deciduous Teeth

right upper	**55 54** *53 52 51*	*61 62* **63 64 65**	left upper
right lower	**85 84** 83 *82 81*	*71 72 73* **74 75**	left lower

Molars <u>Premolars</u> Canines *Incisors*

Figure shows International Classification (F.D.I) of permanent and deciduous teeth.

In *Dental malocclusion* the biting surfaces of the teeth do not properly fit together, which can cause facial and oral pain. The way teeth grow out of the jaw is influenced by several factors, e.g. hereditary conditions or secondary changes in the shape of the jaw (loss of teeth, etc.). If untreated, these variations can lead to problems in biting, oral hygiene and gum health as well as speech.

- **Tongue**

- Examine the **surface of the tongue**. Identify the *body of the tongue, frenulum, median sulcus, sulcus terminalis, foramen cecum* (origin of the thyroglossal duct, from which the thyroid gland develops), *median* and *lateral glossoepiglottic folds*, and the *rt.* and *lt. epiglottic valleculae* on either side of the median glossoepiglottic fold (depression of the spaces between the epiglottis and the dorsal root of the tongue).

- View the **papillae** on the dorsal surface of the tongue: the row of *vallate papillae* anterior and parallel to the sulcus terminalis, the *foliate papillae* laterally, and the *filiform and fungiform papillae* on the remaining dorsal surface of the tongue.

- Identify **different taste regions** on the tongue for salt and sour (*anterolateral 2/3^{rds} of dorsum of tongue*), sweet (*apex of tongue*), and bitter (*region of vallate papillae*).
- Inspect the lymphoid nodules collectively called **lingual tonsil** localised between the *terminal sulcus* and *epiglottis*.
- View the **intrinsic tongue muscles** (superior longitudinal, inferior longitudinal, transverse and vertical muscles), **lingual aponeurosis**, and **extrinsic tongue muscles** (genioglossus, hyoglossus, styloglossus muscles) that are innervated by the *hypoglossal nerve* (CN. XII).
- Localise the sensory **innervation** of the *anterior 2/3^{rds}* (general sensation from lingual nerve from CN. V$_3$, sensation of taste and autonomic innervation from chorda tympani from CN. VII) and the *posterior 1/3rd of the tongue* (general sensation, sensation of taste and autonomic innervation from glossopharyngeal nerve CN. IX).
- View the **blood supply** of the tongue: terminal branch of the lingual artery (supplying the *anterior 2/3^{rds}* of the tongue), and the dorsal lingual artery (supplying the *posterior 1/3rd* of tongue).
- Study the **lymphatic drainage** of the tongue (tip of tongue to submental nodes, *anterolateral 2/3^{rds}* to submandibular nodes, *anteromedial 2/3^{rds}* to deep cervical nodes, the *posterior 1/3rd* of tongue to retropharyngeal nodes).

A restrictive or tight frenulum (*tongue tie*) can impair the ability of the tongue to move. Therefore, it can lead to problems in breastfeeding in newborn babies. If left untreated, a tight frenulum can cause also speech difficulties later.

The *papillae* of the tongue are important for the general sensation and sensation of taste. The posterior 1/3rd of tongue is rough, because the numerous filiform papillae here have a cornified epithelium on their surface (see **Histology** books).

- **Salivary glands**
- View the **three major salivary glands:** The *parotid gland* is totally serous, the *submandibular gland* is seromucous (mostly serous and partially mucous), and the *sublingual gland* is mucoserous (almost completely mucous) (see **Histology**).
- Study **other sources of saliva in the mouth.** The mixed seromucous *anterior lingual gland* (Nuhn) in the lower half of the tongue near the apex, the serous *tubuloacinar glands* (von Ebner) at the bottom of the vallate papillae (anterior to sulcus terminalis on the posterior portion of the tongue), and the mucous *posterior lingual glands* at the dorsum of the tongue.
- Study also secretions produced by mixed mucoserous glands in the *lamina propria* of the *pharynx*, the seromucous glands of the *larynx* (e.g. epiglottis), and the completely mucous glands of the *palate* (pharyngeal, laryngeal and palatine glands).

Components of Saliva	
enzymatic activity:	alpha-amylase, peroxidases
inhibitors of enzymatic activity:	cystatins (proteinase inhibitors)
cleaning of mouth / transport of food:	watery, ions, mucins
	(hydrophilic proteins)
mineralisation of teeth:	ions, pH, statherins, proline-rich proteins
sense of taste:	dissolves substances
protection:	lysozyme, histatins, cystatins, lactoferrin
	sialoperoxidase, IgA antibodies

5.3 BACKGROUND INFORMATION:

- **Branchial (pharyngeal) pouches**

In the Skull-II practical session, we learnt about the branchial (or pharyngeal) arches. The **branchial (pharyngeal) pouches** are lined by the endoderm (see **Embryology** for details) localised between the branchial arches. The structures developing from the branchial pouches are as follows:

- 1st pouch: auditory tube (also pharyngotympanic or Eustachian tube), parts of middle ear, mastoid antrum, and inner layer of the ear drum.

- 2nd pouch: parts of middle ear, palatine tonsils between the palatoglossal and palatopharyngeal arches.

- 3rd pouch: Rt. & lt. inf. parathyroid glands from the dorsal wings and the thymus gland from the ventral wings (fusion of tissue from the rt. & lt. sides). Both structures descend, the inf. parathyroid becoming situated caudal to the sup. glands, and the thymus gland becoming situated in the thorax.

- 4th pouch: Sup. parathyroid glands and thymus gland (same wings as above).

- 5th pouch: Ultimobranchial body, from which the parafollicular C-cells of the thyroid gland develop. They wander in and become incorporated into the thyroid.

- **Branchial (pharyngeal) clefts**

On the ectodermal surface (see **Embryology**), the pharyngeal clefts extend into the gaps between the brachial arches in the neck region to separate them. Disturbances in the development of these clefts in the neck can result in the formation of *lat.* or *med. cervical fistulae* that can be connected with other (abnormal ducts; lat. cervical fistula connected to exterior of the body at site of branchial cleft, med. cervical fistula connected to the interior of the body at the opening of the branchial pouch) or *lat. cervical cysts* (closed sac with its own membrane at site of branchial cleft, usually filled with liquid).

*P.S. Please note that the thyroid gland does <u>not</u> develop from the branchial pouches, but from the **thyroglossal duct**.* Med. & lat. cervical fistula/lat. cervical cysts develop at sites of the branchial pouches/clefts. Therefore, they need to be clearly distinguished from the medi<u>an</u> cervical fistula or cyst, which is a remnant of the thyroglossal duct.

6. INFRATEMPORAL FOSSA, TEMPOROMANDIBULAR JOINT AND MUSCLES OF MASTICATION

In the last session, the zygomatic arch has been removed. This was the first step to **approach the infratemporal fossa**. Today we will further **remove parts** of the **mandible** to open the temporomandibular joint in two ways.

6.1 DISSECTIONS

- **Removal of portions of the mandible**
- **Saw** and remove the **tip of the coronoid process** of the mandible **together with the insertion of the temporalis muscle** and reflect the muscle upwards to its origin at the temporal fossa.
- Clean the bony surface of the coronoid process and ramus of the mandible.
- **Cut out** the **ramus of the mandible** together with the rest of the coronoid process **L-shaped** to access the infratemporal fossa (horizontal saw should cut through the outer plate of the ramus only). **Do not damage the inferior alveolar nerve and its mylohyoid branch here!**

- **Opening of the temporomandibular joint**
- The opening of the temporomandibular joint (TMJ) will be performed **in two ways**:
  1) According to one procedure, the head of the mandible will be **dislocated** from the temporal fossa by opening the capsule of the joint.
  2) According to the second procedure, we will **horizontally saw** a piece of the head of the mandible and the articular tubercle of the temporal bone (ant. to temporal fossa) and the zygomatic process of the temporal bone to see a **section** through the TMJ.

- **Infratemporal fossa**
- Identify the **medial pterygoid muscle** as well as the *superior and inferior heads* of the **lateral pterygoid muscle**.
- Identify the **veins** draining into the *pterygoid venous plexus* before you remove them to continue dissection.
- Find the following **branches of the mandibular nerve** in the infratemporal fossa: *inf. alveolar nerve* with its *mylohyoid branch*, the *lingual nerve* with the *chorda tympani nerve* attached to it, and the *buccal nerve*.
- Find the **branches of the maxillary artery** coursing together with the inferior alveolar nerve and with the motor branches of the mandibular nerve innervating the muscles of mastication.

6.2 PROSECTIONS AND MODELS

- **Bones of the TMJ and muscles of mastication**

- View the bones forming the **zygomatic arch** and their features.

- Study the main features of the **mandible** from the **lateral and medial views**. Identify the *ramus, angle, body, coronoid process, condylar process, head* and *mandibular notch*. View the *mandibular foramen* with the *lingula*, where the mandibular canal starts (for inferior alveolar nerve), and the *mental foramen*. Find the *mylohyoid line*, and identify the borders of the *sublingual fossa* above and the *digastric fossa* and *submandibular fossa* below this line for the origins of suprahyoid muscles involved in opening of mouth and chewing. Find the mental spine (origin of genioglossus and geniohyoid muscles) and mental protuberance.

- Identify, **parts of the temporal bone** related to the **temporomandibular joint (TMJ)** (*mandibular fossa*, the *articular eminence* at the zygomatic process of the temporal bone, *petrotympanic* and *squamatympanic fissures*) and *attachments of the temporalis muscle* (temporal fossa, superior & inferior temporal lines).

- Identify the **origins and insertions** of the three other **muscles of mastication** innervated by the *mandibular nerve* (masseter, med. and lat. pterygoids).

- Identify the **origins and insertions** of **muscles of facial expression** required for opening and closing of the mouth, and the buccinator muscle.

- Inspect the *two compartments*, the *articular surfaces* and *ligaments* of the **TMJ** with their attachments to the skull and mandible. Discuss the **movements of the mandible** (protrusion, retraction, elevation, depression).

Temporomandibular (joint) disorders involve the *jaw joints, the muscles that control jaw movement*, and *dental occlusion*. The *imbalance* in movements of the jaw and skull (articular surfaces, ligaments & muscles) can result in *muscle fatigue and spasms, joint dysfunction*, and also in *changes in the teeth*. **Symptoms** can also include headache, pain (facial, jaw, ear and/or neck), restricted mouth opening, difficulties in chewing, clenching of teeth, dizziness and tinnitus (sound in the ear despite absence of corresponding external sounds). Therefore, patients with these disorders are *often classified as chronic pain patients*.

- **Muscles of mastication, infratemporal fossa and maxillary artery**

- Recall the *borders of the infratemporal fossa* (**see Practical Session Skull-II**).

- View the *muscles, blood vessels* and *nerves* in the **infratemporal fossa** as described above (med. & lat. pterygoid muscles, maxillary artery, venous pterygoid plexus, proximal portion of the mandibular nerve, lingual nerve with chorda tympani nerve, inferior alveolar nerve with mylohyoid nerve). You will not see the med. & lat. pterygoid muscles before the zygomatic arch is removed and the masseter muscle is reflected, because they are hidden in the infratemporal fossa.

- Inspect the **four main muscles of mastication** supplied by *branches of the mandibular nerve* and the *maxillary artery* closer: the masseter, temporalis, and med. & lat. pterygoid muscles. Name their origins and insertions, and function.

- Name the **branches of the maxillary artery**. These include arteries supplying the cheek (*buccal*), meninges (*middle meningeal*), auricular region (*deep auricular, anterior tympanic*) and the palate (*descending palatine*). Other arteries accompany the branches of the mandibular (*deep temporal, med. & lateral pterygoid & masseteric* to muscles of mastication, *inferior alveolar* to lower teeth), and maxillary nerves (*infraorbital, greater and lesser palatine, nasopalatine*). The *sphenopalatine artery* is the end branch entering the nasal cavity.

- **Trigeminal nerve**

Study in detail the branches of the **3 divisions of the trigeminal nerve** on their course from the skull base to their targets:

- The **first division**, the **ophthalmic nerve (CN. V$_1$)**, which is **entirely sensory**, enters the orbit through the *superior orbital fissure*. Its branches are the *frontal* (supraorbital & supratrochlear branches), *nasociliary* (ant. & post. ethmoidal branches, short & long ciliary branches), *lacrimal* and *tentorial nerves*.

- The **second division** of the trigeminal nerve, the **maxillary nerve (CN. V$_2$)**, also has **sensory fibres only**. It enters the *pterygopalatine fossa* through the *foramen rotundum*, where it gives rise to the following branches: the *infraorbital nerve* (with the post., middle & ant. sup. alveolar branches), *zygomatic nerve* (zygomaticotemporal & zygomaticofacial branches), and the *greater and lesser palatine, posterolateral nasal, nasopalatine* (long sphenopalatine), and *meningeal nerves*.

- The **third division**, the **mandibular nerve (CN. V$_3$)**, has **both sensory and motor components**. It enters the *infratemporal fossa* through the *foramen ovale*. Its sensory branches are the *lingual nerve* (joins the chorda tympani nerve), *inf. alveolar nerve* (inferior alveolar plexus, mental nerve with incisive branch) *except its mylohyoid branch*, and the *auriculotemporal, buccal & meningeal nerves*. The mandibular nerve is the only division of the trigeminal nerve sending off direct *motor branches* (see below).

The **trigeminal nerve** is an entirely sensory nerve except its mandibular division, which has both motor and sensory components. The mandibular division carrying motor fibres (radix motoria) innervates the **muscles of mastication** (masseter, temporalis, med. and lat. pterygoids), *tensor tympani* and *tensor veli palatini muscles,* and *two muscles at the floor of the mouth* (anterior belly of the digastric & mylohyoid muscles).

In a **broader sense**, some *muscles of facial expression* that are innervated by the *facial nerve*, and *suprahyoid muscles* involved in chewing and movements of the mandible can also be regarded as **muscles of mastication** (see **Anterior Neck Practical**).

The sensory afferents of the trigeminal nerve also transmit **pain**, e.g. pain induced by dental caries (generalised pain), pulpitis (localised pain), infected salivary glands, etc. "Tooth ache" can also be mimicked by a lesion or inflammation at more proximal parts of the maxillary or mandibular nerves (parts of the nerve closer to the brainstem) not related to the teeth, e.g. trigeminal neuralgia or sinusitis in the maxillary air sinus, called **referred pain**. If misdiagnosed, this can even lead to extraction of teeth. Pain in the *temporomandibular joint* can be referred to the *ear*, because the auriculotemporal nerve provides the sensory innervation of both the joint and the auricle.

The site of the lesion causing pain may also be localised in the central nervous system (cortex, nuclei, and tracts). This phenomenon is called **central pain**.

7. ANTERIOR NECK REGION

In the anterior neck region, we have **already dissected** the *platysma* and some *superficial blood vessels and nerves* (e.g. transverse cervical vein and nerve, superficial cervical ansa). While doing so we have also removed the *superficial cervical fascia of the neck*. However, the **deep cervical fascia** has many components that should have remained intact. Today we will dissect the *cutaneous branches of the cervical plexus*, and *remove fascial coverings* in the anterior neck region **except the prevertebral layer** of the deep cervical fascia. This will allow us to find the *hypoglossal* and *phrenic nerves* in the anterior neck region.

7.1 DISSECTIONS

- **Cutaneous branches of cervical plexus & accessory nerve (CN. XI)**
- Identify the so-called **nerve point** (or *punctum nervosum*) at the posterolateral border of the sternocleidomastoid muscle, where we have already dissected the *transverse cervical nerve* and its anastomosis with the *cervical branch of the facial nerve* (*superficial cervical ansa*). Make sure that the platysma has been lifted, and reflected cranially.
- Now dissect all other **cutaneous branches of the cervical plexus**, which are called the *lesser occipital, great auricular, transverse cervical*, and *supraclavicular nerves* (with lateral, intermediate & medial branches).
- Find the *trapezius muscle* and the **accessory nerve** coursing in cranio-caudal direction at the medial edge of the muscle.

- **Fascial coverings**
- We have already removed the superficial cervical fascia below the skin. Now remove carefully the *investing fascia*, which is *part of the deep fascia of the neck*, and envelops the *sternocleidomastoid muscle*. **Do not damage the branches of the cervical plexus!**
- Remove the anterior portion of the *visceral fascia*, and dissect the *infrahyoid muscles*, which are the *sternohyoid, sternothyroid, thyrohyoid* and *omohyoid muscles*. **Do not open the carotid sheath!**
- Next dissect at the **posterior aspect of the floor of the mouth** the *stylohyoid muscle*, and *posterior belly of the digastric muscle* by removing their fascia
- Now remove at the **anterior aspect of the floor of the mouth** the fascia of the *mylohyoid muscle* and *anterior belly of the digastric muscle*.
- Identify the *deep cervical ansa* forming a loop above the *carotid sheath* and attachment of the *tendon of the omohyoid muscle* to the carotid sheath. By stretching the carotid sheath, the omohyoid muscle keeps the lumen of the *internal jugular vein* open. **Do not damage the deep cervical ansa!**

- **Hypoglossal nerve and deep cervical ansa**
- Dissect the **hypoglossal nerve** (CN. XII) in the submandibular triangle.
- Find the **sup. (ant.) root** of the *deep ansa cervicalis (profunda)* at that point, where it leaves the hypoglossal nerve (CN. XII).
- Dissect the **loop** of the *deep ansa cervicalis* formed by the *sup. (ant.)* and *inf. (post.) roots*, the latter coming from **motor branches of the cervical plexus**. The loop of the ansa cervicalis should be attached to the outer surface of the *carotid sheath*.
- Dissect branches of the *deep ansa cervicalis* coursing to and innervating the **infrahyoid muscles**.

- **Phrenic nerve**
- Find the **ant. scalene muscle** by first localising the *subclavian vein*, which courses anterior to the muscle and then the *subclavian artery*, which courses between the ant. and middle scalene muscles.
- Dissect the **phrenic nerve** on the *ant. scalene muscle* (leading muscle for identification) on its course from the neck to the thorax.
- During dissections you may also encounter the *brachial plexus*, which passes through the space between the ant. and middle scalene muscles on its way to the axilla.

The **fascial coverings of the neck** can be divided into a *superficial cervical fascia* and *deep cervical fascia*. The deep cervical fascia has several layers as listed below:

(i) The *investing fascia* covers the *sternocleidomastoid muscle*.

(ii) The *visceral fascia* (pretracheal & buccopharyngeal components) surrounds the *four infrahyoid muscles* and *visceral organs of the neck* (thyroid gland and parathyroid glands, above C6 pharynx, below C6 larynx or oesophagus / trachea).

The posterior part of the visceral fascia (*buccopharyngeal component*) is stretched between the rt. and lt. *carotid sheaths* (each sheath contains the respective *common carotid artery, internal jugular vein* and *vagus nerve*).

(iii) The *prevertebral fascia* surrounds the *vertebral column* (including the seven cervical vertebrae, eight pairs of spinal nerves from C1-C8, and cervical spinal cord) and *autochtone back muscles* (ant. vertebral muscles flexing the neck, post. vertebral muscles extending the neck). Furthermore, the prevertebral fascia is in continuity with the axillary sheath.

The **space** between the visceral fascia (posterior part or buccopharyngeal component) and prevertebral fascia is called the *retropharyngeal space*. The retropharyngeal space is further subdivided by the *alar fascia* into anterior and posterior portions. The posterior portion contains the cervical sympathetic trunk with the superior, middle and inferior cervical sympathetic ganglia.

The retropharyngeal space extends laterally, where it is called *lateropharyngeal* space coming into close contact with the palatine tonsil and parotid gland.

7.2 PROSECTIONS AND MODELS

- **Anterior triangle of the neck**

- View the *anterior triangle* of the neck between the *mandible, midline of the anterior neck* and the *anterior border of the sternocleidomastoid muscle*.

- Now view the **four subdivisions** of the anterior triangle of the neck with their contents:

    1) Find the borders of the *lt.* and *rt.* **submandibular triangle** between the *mandible*, and *anterior* and *posterior bellies of the digastric muscle*.

    View the *contents* of the triangle, which are the submandibular gland, the lingual and facial arteries, the mylohyoid nerve (from CN. V_3), the hypoglossal nerve (CN. XII), and the submandibular lymph nodes.

    2) Find the borders of the *lt.* and *rt.* **carotid triangle** between the *posterior belly of the digastric muscle, anterior border of the sternocleidomastoid muscle*, and *superior belly of the omohyoid muscle*.

    View the *contents* of the triangle. These are the common carotid artery and internal jugular vein with their branches, the branch of the *glossopharyngeal nerve* (CN. IX) to the *carotid body* (glomus caroticum) situated at the bifurcation of the common carotid artery, the *vagus nerve* (CN. X) coursing in the carotid sheath, deep cervical lymph nodes, and the *hypoglossal nerve* (CN. XII) before it ascends to the submandibular triangle.

    3) Find the borders of the unpaired **submental triangle**, between the *lt.* and *rt. anterior bellies of the digastric muscles* and the *hyoid bone*.

    4) Find the borders of the *lt.* and *rt.* **muscular triangle** between the *midline of the anterior neck*, and the *superior belly of the omohyoid muscle* and the *anterior border of the sternocleidomastoid muscle*.

- **Floor of the mouth (suprahyoid muscles)**

View the **suprahyoid muscles**, which contribute to mastication by depressing the mandible, if the hyoid bone is kept fixed by activation of the infrahyoid muscles. Therefore, they can be regarded as muscles of mastication in a broader sense.

- The *anterior belly of the digastric muscle* and the *mylohyoid* muscle innervated by the **mylohyoid nerve** (from the inferior alveolar nerve from the mandibular nerve CN. V_3).

- The *posterior belly of the digastric muscle* and the *stylohyoid muscle* innervated by the **facial nerve** (CN. VII).

- The *geniohyoid muscle* innervated by the **hypoglossal nerve** (CN. XII).

- **Infrahyoid (strap) muscles**
- View the *four infrahyoid muscles* that lie in front of the larynx, which are also called strap muscles. They are the *sternohyoid, sternothyroid, thyrohyoid,* and *omohyoid muscles.*
- You have learned about their innervation today, when you have dissected the *deep cervical ansa.*

- **Course of phrenic nerve**
- View the phrenic nerve in the **neck** on the anterior scalene muscle.
- Follow the course of the phrenic nerve through the **superior thoracic aperture**.
- Inspect the phrenic nerve in the **thorax**, where it provides the sensory innervation to the *parietal pleura* (mediastinal and diaphragmatic parts) and *pericardial sac* as well as the motor innervation to the *diaphragm*.
- View the *phrenicoabdominal branch* of the phrenic nerve **passing through the diaphragm** (*left*: through caval opening for inf. vena cava, *right*: through oesophageal hiatus) to provide the sensory innervation of some parts of the *peritoneum* in the **upper abdomen**.

The **phrenic nerve** originating from the cervical segments C3-C5 (mainly C4) innervates structures located much more caudally. Some background information may be useful to understand this phenomenon. During development structures innervated by the phrenic nerve *descend* together with the nerve. These are the pericardium (from the pleurapericardial membrane) containing the heart and diaphragm (from the pleuroperitoneal membrane / septum transversum), which later separate the intraembryonic coelom into three types of cavities: the pericardial cavity, lt. and rt. pleural cavities (from primitive pleural cavity), and peritoneal cavity. For this reason, the phrenic nerve also supplies some parts of the peritoneum in the upper abdomen with a sensory innervation, and gall stones cause pain in the shoulder. This is another example for referred pain (sensory innervation of the shoulder from C5, the shoulder is the Head's zone for the gall bladder).

Therefore, lesions of the neck damaging either the phrenic nerve, the cervical spinal cord at C3-C4 or higher, or the roots of cervical spinal nerves C3-C5 can paralyse the diaphragm, which is the major muscle required for **inspiration**.

8. DEEP CERVICAL REGION AND THE SUBMANDIBULAR GANGLION

We will continue neck dissection as described in the last practical session by focusing on two regions in today's session. First, we will **open the carotid sheath**, find the vagus nerve in the sheath, and dissect all branches of the external carotid artery. Next, we will dissect the **lingual nerve** to demonstrate its whole course from the infratemporal fossa to the submandibular region and oral cavity, and will find the **submandibular ganglion**.

8.1 DISSECTIONS

- **Opening of the carotid sheath**

- <u>Do not damage the **deep cervical ansa**</u> when you open the *carotid sheath*.

- **Within the carotid sheath**, you will find the *common carotid artery* medially (!). The *internal jugular vein* lies lateral to the artery in the neck. Carefully remove the loose irregular connective tissue between the vessels using tweezers, and expose the *vagus nerve (CN. X)*.

- Next, you can remove the entire carotid sheath. Thereby you may also open lateral portions of the *alar fascia* and/or *prevertebral layer of the (deep) cervical fascia*.

- You should take your class mate's / colleague's **carotid pulse** since this is often done to check if a person is still living. Feel the *common carotid artery* in the *carotid triangle* lateral to the thyroid cartilage. **But touch the carotid artery gently**, because stimulating the baroreceptors in the *carotid sinus* by vigorous palpation (touching) can provoke **severe bradycardia** or **even stop the heart** in some sensitive persons. Also, a person's <u>two carotid arteries should never be palpated at the same time</u> to avoid a risk of fainting or brain ischemia.

- View the **surface markings of the internal jugular vein**. The internal jugular vein lies posterior to the internal carotid artery in the uppermost part of its course after leaving the jugular foramen of the skull. In the middle of the neck, the vein comes to lie laterally. Thus, the surface projection of the internal jugular vein is represented by a line from the *ear lobule* to the *medial end of the clavicle*. The position of the vein can also be identified by palpating the common carotid artery, because the vein lies lateral to the artery (e.g. before cannulation of the vein for placing a central venous catheter).

- **External carotid artery**

- Find the **bifurcation of the common carotid artery** at the vertebral levels C3-C5 and then dissect all branches of the external carotid artery.

1) The **first anterior branch** of the external carotid artery will be the *sup. thyroid artery* giving rise to the *sup. laryngeal artery*, which divides into an *external* and *internal branch*. The **two other anterior branches** are the *lingual* and *facial arteries*.

CAUTION: The *sup. laryngeal artery* will lead you to the *thyrohyoid membrane*. At the membrane, the artery courses together with the *superior laryngeal nerve* and perforates the membrane together with the *internal branch* of the *superior laryngeal nerve*.

Do not damage the superior laryngeal nerve when dissecting the sup. laryngeal artery!

2) The **middle branch** of external carotid artery is the *ascending pharyngeal artery*.

3) The **two posterior branches** of external carotid artery are the *occipital* and *posterior auricular arteries*.

4) The **two end branches** of external carotid artery are the *superficial temporal* and *maxillary arteries*.

- **Lingual nerve and submandibular ganglion at the floor of the mouth**

- After the dissection steps described above, you can now identify in the **submandibular triangle** the *submandibular gland*, and the *lingual* and *facial arteries*.

- Dissect the *mylohyoid nerve* (from inferior alveolar nerve from CN. V3) coursing upon the mylohyoid muscle in the submandibular triangle.

- **Cut** the *anterior belly of the digastric muscle* and the *mylohyoid muscle* **at the margin of the mandible** and reflect them laterally and inferiorly.

- Now you can dissect the **lingual nerve** and find the **submandibular ganglion**, which is connected through *preganglionic* and *postganglionic fibres* coursing between the lingual nerve and ganglion.

- **Course of the lingual nerve in the oral cavity**

- **Cannulate the ducts** of the three salivary glands - a procedure used for sialography (radiography of the glands), e.g. to detect a calcified deposit (sialolith) in a duct.

- **Remove the mucosa** at the inferior surface of the tongue up to the root of the tongue. This is necessary to dissect the *lingual nerve* (from CN. V3) and the submandibular duct. But **preserve the mucosa** at the **opening of the duct**.

- Dissect the lingual nerve coursing from laterally at around the 3rd lower molar, and lateral edge of the hyoglossus muscle towards medially, where it **undercrosses the submandibular duct** (runs **below the duct**), and reaches the tip of the tongue.

8.2 PROSECTIONS AND MODELS

- **Identify the structures dissected in today's practical session**
- Branches of the external carotid artery.
- The inferior alveolar nerve and mylohyoid nerve.
- Lingual nerve in the submandibular triangle & oral cavity, submandibular ganglion.

- **Course of the vagus nerve**
- Inspect the course of the *vagus nerve* in the **neck** between the common carotid artery and internal jugular vein. Find the *superior laryngeal nerve*, which is a branch of the vagus nerve.
- Follow the course of the *rt. and lt. vagus nerves* in the **thorax**. Find the *right recurrent laryngeal nerve* turning upward around the rt. subclavian artery and the *left recurrent laryngeal nerve* around the aortic arch. View the *oesophagus* with the ant. and post. vagal plexus.
- Learn about the course of the branches of the vagus nerve in the **abdomen**, e.g. along the small curvature of the stomach **(see Abdomen session)**.

- **Thyroid and parathyroid glands**
- Inspect the **divisions of the thyroid gland**: *Rt.* and *lt. lobes* (reaching to the pharyngeal constrictors and oesophagus posteriorly) connected by the *isthmus* above the trachea. Find also the *pyramidal lobe* (present in 50 % of cases) corresponding to thyroid gland tissue extending cranially from the isthmus. It develops out of the *thyroglossal duct* along its course during development (before bifurcation of glandular tissue into rt. and lt. lobes). Thyroid gland tissue can even develop at the *base of the tongue*, as the thyroglossal duct has its origin at the *foramen cecum of the tongue*.
- View the **recurrent laryngeal nerve** coursing in the *crevice* between the oesophagus and posterior part of the thyroid gland, where it can be damaged during surgery of the thyroid gland.
- View the **arterial blood supply** of the thyroid gland from the *superior thyroid artery* (from external carotid artery) and *inferior thyroid artery* (branch of thyrocervical trunk arising from the subclavian artery).
- View the **venous drainage** via the *superior and middle thyroid veins* draining into the internal jugular vein and *inferior thyroid vein* draining into the brachiocephalic trunk.
- Identify the four **parathyroid glands** (two on each side) embedded within the *posterior capsule* of the thyroid gland. If they are accidentally removed during thyroidectomy together with the thyroid gland, the patient will suffer from *hypocalcaemia* (see below).

The thyroid and parathyroid glands are **endocrine glands**. The *thyroid gland* produces the **thyroid hormones** *thyroxin* (T4) *and triiodothyronine* (T3) incorporated in a larger protein (*thyroglobulin*). Thyroglobulin is stored in the colloid in *follicles*. It is degraded if required to release of T3 & T4 into the blood stream to enhance metabolism (upon stimulation with the thyroid stimulating hormone TSH).

The *C-cells* of the thyroid gland (originate from ultimobranchial body at the 5th branchial pouch) produce **calcitonin**, which is an **antagonist** of **parathyroid hormone**. Parathyroid hormone mobilises calcium from bone (gross regulation), whereas calcitonin supports calcium uptake into the bone (fine tuning).

An enlarged thyroid gland called **struma** (also goitre) will lead to a swelling in the neck (lateral lobes, isthmus, pyramidal lobe) just below the thyroid cartilage, the largest and most prominent cartilage of the larynx **(Adam's apple)**. A struma can lead to disturbances in breathing and swallowing. If a patient has a struma, **accessory thyroid gland tissue** localised along the track of the degenerated thyroglossal duct will also enlarge, e.g. resulting in a *retrolingual struma* (or goitre). Note that a struma can be associated either with hypo- or with hyperthyroidism.

9. BACK OF THE NECK

Muscles, nerves and vessels in the **posterior neck**, and their **extension to the head** region will be studied.

9.1 DISSECTIONS

- **Occipital artery and greater occipital nerve**
- First clean the subcutaneous fatty and connective tissue, which was left after removing the skin.
- Thereby, **you have to pay particular attention to the preservation of** the *occipital artery* coursing together with the *greater occipital nerve* (posterior ramus of C2). This can be a challenging task, because the subcutaneous fatty and connective tissue will be quite compact.
- You may also find the *3rd occipital nerve* (posterior ramus of C3).

- **Trapezius muscle**
- Mobilise the *trapezius muscle* **bluntly** from underlying muscles.
- Now cut the trapezius muscle off at its *origin* at the *occipital bone* (supreme nuchal line and external occipital protuberance), as well as at the *nuchal ligament.*
- Finally, reflect the muscle laterally and find the **accessory nerve** and *cervical motor branches* sending off branches to the trapezius and sternocleidomastoid muscles.

- **Autochtone (intrinsic) back muscles**
- Next you will have mobilise the *splenius capitis* muscle **bluntly** from underlying muscles, before you cut off the muscle at its *insertion* (!) at the *superior nuchal line* and *mastoid process* (the insertion point laterally). Reflect the splenius capitis muscle laterally.
- Now you will see the *semispinalis capitis muscle* lying under the splenius capitis muscle. Mobilise the semispinalis capitis muscle **bluntly** and cut it off at its *insertion* (!) just below the *superior nuchal line* and the *spinous processes of the cervical vertebrae* (!). Reflect the muscle laterally.

- **Short nuchal muscles and suboccipital triangle**
- Find the **short nuchal muscles** (deep nuchal muscles), which are bounded by a *common fascia*. They are the *rectus capitis posterior major, rectus capitis posterior minor, obliquus capitis superior and obliquus capitis inferior muscles.*

- Identify the **suboccipital triangle** formed by the *rectus capitis posterior major, obliquus capitis superior* and *obliquus capitis inferior muscles.*
- Dissect the **floor** of the triangle to find the **vertebral artery.** It is formed by the *posterior occipito-atlantal membrane*, and the *posterior arch of the atlas*, upon which you will find the artery after it has left the *transverse foramina* of the cervical vertebrae and before it enters the intracranial cavity through the *foramen magnum.*
- Find the **first cervical** (*suboccipital nerve*) in the deep groove on the upper surface of the posterior arch of the atlas next to the vertebral artery.

9.2 PROSECTIONS AND MODELS

- **Posterior triangle of the neck**
- View the **posterior triangle** of the neck between the *posterior border of the sternocleidomastoid muscle, anterior border of the trapezius muscle* and the *clavicle.*
- About 2.5 cm above the clavicle, it is **subdivided** by the *inferior belly* of the *omohyoid muscle* **into two more triangles**: the larger *occipital* and the smaller *subclavian (omoclavicular) triangles.*

- **Vertebral artery (extracranial course)**
- View the course of the **vertebral artery** within the transverse foramina of the cervical vertebrae, and in the suboccipital triangle, where it courses on the posterior arch of the atlas before it penetrates the atlantooccipital membrane.

- **Epicranius muscle and epicranial aponeurosis**
- View the two bellies of the **occipitofrontal** (*epicranius*) muscle. The *frontal* and *occipital bellies* of the muscle are connected by the **galea aponeurotica** (epicranial aponeurosis).

A **subgaleal (subaponeurotic) haematoma** results from blood accumulation in the *"subgaleal space"* between the *galea aponeurotica* and *periosteum of the skull* (pericranium) following a rupture of *emissary veins*. Because the haemorrhage is not limited by the suture lines of the skull, a subgaleal haemorrhage can acquire a considerable volume. It can extend forward to the orbital margins, backward to the nuchal ridge and laterally to the temporal fascia resulting in severe hypovolaemia (e.g. in new born babies or skull fractures).

In contrast a **cephalhaematoma** is a **subperiosteal haemorrhage** in the *"subperiosteal space"* between the periosteum and the naked skull bone that is *confined by suture lines* because of the periosteal attachment. Therefore, it is less dangerous than a subgaleal haematoma.

- **Venous drainage of the head and neck**

The veins of the head and neck may be **subdivided into** (i) veins of the exterior of the head and face, (ii), the veins of the brain and skull, and (iii) the veins of the neck.

(i) On the exterior of the head and face, find the *facial vein* (with the *angular vein* draining into it), *superficial temporal vein, pterygoid plexus, maxillary vein, retromandibular vein* (with its anterior and posterior divisions), *common facial vein, posterior auricular vein*, and the *occipital vein*.

(ii) Recapitulate the *venous dural sinuses, diploic veins* and *emissary veins* draining the brain and skull (see **Neuroanatomy** for veins of the brain).

(iii) View the veins of the neck, which return the blood from the head and face: these are the external jugular, anterior jugular, internal jugular, and vertebral veins.

The **anastomoses** between the **veins of the face and skull** are important for spreading of infections and malignant tumours. E.g. the *pterygoid plexus* (drains into the *maxillary vein*) connects the *facial vein* through an **emissary vein** to the *cavernous sinus*. The **pterygoid plexus** itself drains the *inferior ophthalmic, infraorbital, sphenopalatine, deep facial, palatine, inferior alveolar, muscular* (from muscles of mastication) and *buccal veins*. Therefore, the pterygoid plexus holds a **key position** in linking many anterior facial regions with the intracranial cavity, which can result in a **cavernous sinus thrombosis** if infections are carried forward.

The **veins of the orbit** also play a key role in connecting the *retromandibular* and *facial veins* with venous dural sinuses (cavernous sinus). *Such anastomoses* are found between (i) the frontal branch of the superficial temporal vein and supraorbital/supratrochlear veins; (ii) the transverse facial vein and inferior palpaebral veins; and (iii) between the angular vein and dorsal nasal vein/supratrochlear vein (for further examples of intracranial/extracranial venous connections see **Skull-II Practical**).

- **Lymphatic drainage of the head and neck**

- View the location of *occipital, postauricular* (mastoid), *preauricular* (superficial and deep parotid), *submandibular, submental, deep cervical, retropharyngeal* and *jugulodigastric lymph nodes*, and the *deep cervical chain of lymph nodes*.

- **Mark the positions of lymph node groups** on the head & neck of a <u>student in your group</u> with colours used for face painting. Use different colours for **deep** and **superficial** lymph nodes.

- Now learn to **palpate them** in a sequence and discuss the **structures they drain**.

10. PHARYNX, LARYNX AND SUPRA-CLAVICULAR FOSSA

In this practical session, we will **complete** the **dissection of the neck region**.

10.1 DISSECTIONS

- **Retropharyngeal space and cervical sympathetic trunk**

- Posterior to the inlets of the carotid sheath you will find the *alar fascia*, which is localised in the retropharyngeal space. The retropharyngeal space is localised between the pharynx and prevertebral muscles, which are covered by the *buccopharyngeal fascia* (posterior part of the visceral fascia) and *prevertebral layer of the (deep) cervical fascia*, respectively.

- Now open the whole retropharyngeal space **bluntly** from two sides (on the left and the right). Inspect the *three pharyngeal constrictor muscles*.

- Remove the *alar fascia*, and reveal the **cervical sympathetic trunk** in the retropharyngeal space hidden behind the alar fascia.

- Dissect the *superior*, *middle* and *inferior cervical* **sympathetic ganglia**. The inferior ganglion is usually fused with the first thoracic sympathetic ganglion (T1) to form the *stellate ganglion*.

A **complex regional pain syndrome (CRPS)** is a condition usually affecting *one limb,* and here preferably *the hand or foot*. The key symptom of CRPS is enduring heavy pain that can spread to the entire limb. Typically the pain is out of proportion to the severity of the injury if an injury can be identified. Other typical features include alterations in the *temperature & color of the skin* (mostly flushing, rubor or paleness) accompanied by *intense burning pain, sweating* and *swelling.* The symptoms often deteriorate over time if not treated. Motor symptoms and muscular damage can accompany the other symptoms, and in severe cases this can even lead to contractures.

The origin of CRPS is unknown, but it is thought that the **sympathetic nervous system** plays an important role in generating the symptoms and sustaining the pain. Alternatively, CRPS may be induced by an immune response resulting in typical inflammatory symptoms, i.e. redness, warmth, and swelling.

Therefore, one treatment of CRPS is a **sympathetic nerve block** (e.g. blockade of the stellate ganglion) in addition to other therapies aimed at relieving pain (topical analgesics, antidepressants, corticosteroids, and opioids) or physiotherapy.

- **Superior and inferior laryngeal nerves**

- During dissection of the branches of the *external carotid artery* we have found the *sup. laryngeal artery* (from sup. thyroid artery*)*, which sends off a branch perforating the thyrohyoid membrane together with the **internal branch** of the **superior laryngeal nerve**. Here, we could also see the **external branches** of the artery and nerve.

- Now **trace back** the *internal and external branches* of the superior laryngeal nerve to find the **main trunk** of the nerve and dissect it cranially until you find the point, where the *superior laryngeal nerve* branches off from the **vagus nerve** (CN. X).

- To find the *recurrent laryngeal nerve* **bluntly** open the lt. and rt. crevices lateral to the trachea, and separate the nerve from the surrounding connective tissue.

- Now dissect the **inferior laryngeal nerve** innervating the larynx, which is the _end branch_ of the *recurrent laryngeal nerve*, on the dorsal surface of the lateral lobes of the thyroid gland.

- **Subclavian artery**

- Dissect the **vertebral artery** and **thyrocervical trunk**, the **first two branches** of the subclavian artery coursing cranially.

- Find the **branches** of the *thyrocervical trunk*, which are the *inferior thyroid, transverse cervical* and *suprascapular arteries*. The *ascending cervical artery* is usually a branch of the inferior thyroid artery.

- Identify the **internal thoracic artery** coursing caudally and giving rise to *anterior intercostal arteries*.

- Dissect the **costocervical trunk** with the following two branches: *deep cervical artery* and *supreme intercostal artery*.

- **Brachial plexus in the neck**

- Expose the *brachial plexus* providing the nerve supply of the arm supraclavicularly by gently removing the fatty tissue in the **supraclavicular groove**.

- **Do not damage** the *branches of the subclavian artery* and the *omohyoid muscle* coursing posteriorly on its way to its insertion at the scapula.

- Dissect the **trunks** and **supraclavicular branches** of the *brachial plexus*.

- Continue dissection of the **cords** of the *brachial plexus* **below the clavicle** and in the **axilla** together with axillary vessels (if time is left).

10.2 PROSECTIONS AND MODELS

- **Naso-, oro- and laryngopharynx**

- The **nasopharynx** is the superior division of the pharynx lying above the soft palate/uvula. It communicates with the *auditory tube* (also called pharyngotympanic or Eustachian tube) and *nasal cavity* (through choanae). It contains the *pharyngeal tonsil* (adenoids), *salpingopharyngeal fold*, and *pharyngeal recess*. The opening of the auditory tube lies between the *torus tubarius* (cartilage of the auditory tube below the mucosa) and an elevation called *torus levatorius* evoked by the *levator veli palatini muscle*.

- The **oropharynx** reaches from the soft palate to the root of the tongue and/or to the epiglottis. It communicates with the nasopharynx and oral cavity through the fauces (isthmus faucium). It contains the *palatine tonsil* lying between the *palatoglossal* and *palatopharyngeal arches* (formed by the homonymous muscles).

- The **laryngopharynx** reaches from the root of the tongue/epiglottis to the entrance of the oesophagus at C6. It communicates with the oropharynx and larynx. It contains the *epiglottis, glossoepiglottic folds, valleculae*, and *piriform recess*.

- Identify the *superior, middle* and *inferior* **pharyngeal constrictor muscles** with their origins, and their insertion at the *pharyngeal raphe*. Study the base of the skull and trace the attachments of the pharynx at the inferior aspect of the skull base. Find the *laryngeal gaps*.

- View the *palatopharyngeus* and *stylopharyngeus muscles*, which are the **pharyngeal elevators** (longitudinal muscles of the pharynx).

- View the course of the *glossopharyngeal nerve* (CN. IX) on the *stylopharyngeus muscle*. The nerve supply to the pharynx is provided by a **nervous plexus** formed by the **glossopharyngeal** and **vagus nerves**. Nevertheless, the **motor innervation** originates largely from fibres coming from the cranial root of the accessory nerve (CN. XI), which course together with the *vagus nerve* (CN. X), whereas the **sensory innervation** is mainly from the *glossopharyngeal nerve*. Thus, the accessory nerve supplies the pharyngeal constrictors and the palatopharyngeus muscle, and the glossopharyngeal nerve supplies the stylopharyngeus muscle.

If tonsillar crypts get blocked in tonsillitis, this may lead to **tonsillar pus pockets**. A **peritonsillar abscess** (*quinsy*) is a complication of tonsillitis formed by an accumulation of pus in the peritonsillar region. The abscess can *penetrate the fascia* of the pharyngeal constrictors and spread within the *lateropharyngeal space*. The lateropharyngeal space is the lateral extension of the *retropharyngeal space* coming into close contact with the ramus of the mandible and parotid gland.

- **Cartilaginous and bony skeleton of the larynx**

- Inspect the **hyoid bone** with the *corpus*, and *rt. & lt. cornu minus* and *rt. & lt. cornu majus*. It is a *free-floating bone* embedded between the suprahyoid and infrahyoid muscles. **Note** that the *middle pharyngeal constrictor* has its origin, and the *pharyngeal elevators* have their insertions at the hyoid bone.

- Study the characteristics of the **unpaired** *thyroid*, and *cricoid cartilages* and of the *epiglottis*.

- Study the characteristics of the **paired cartilages** of the larynx (arytenoid cartilages, corniculate cartilages, cuneiform cartilages)
- Inspect the *cricothyroid* and *cricoarytenoid* **joints**.
- Find the *thyrohyoid membrane, cricothyroid ligament* and *cricothyroid membrane*, which are the **external ligaments** of the larynx as well as the *vocal ligaments* and *ventricular ligaments* (false vocal folds), which are **internal ligaments** of the larynx. View also the *aryepiglottic ligaments* and the *quadrangular membrane*.

- **Laryngeal inlet (aditus) and sensory innervation**
- Inspect the **lumen of the larynx**. First, delineate the *vestibule* reaching from the *ventricular (or vestibular) folds* to the entrance of the larynx at the level of the hyoid bone. Next, find the *ventricle* between the upper *ventricular folds* and lower *vocal folds*, and the *laryngeal saccule*, which is a blind pouch extending upward from the ventricle. Finally, inspect the *infraglottic cavity* below the vocal folds.
- Inspect the *palatoglossal* and *palatopharyngeal arches* and the relation of the *root* of the *tongue* to the *epiglottis*, the *piriform recess*, and *aryepiglottic folds*.
- Distinguish the **true** vocal folds (or cords) from the **false** folds (ventricular or vestibular fold), and view the **two divisions of the vocal folds**, which can be **closed separately** once the vocal folds have been opened: the *intermembranous part* (pars intermembranacea) lying anteriorly, and the *intercartilaginous part* between the two arytenoid cartilages lying posteriorly (pars intercartilaginea).
- Find the *internal branch* of the *superior laryngeal nerve*, supplying the **mucosa** of the larynx **above the vocal cords**, and the *inferior laryngeal nerve* (terminal segment of the recurrent laryngeal nerve after it has given off branches to the trachea, oesophagus, thyroid gland and inferior constrictor muscle) innervating the mucosa **below the vocal cords**.

- **Muscles of the larynx and motor innervation**
- Name the **extrinsic muscles** of the larynx, which belong to the muscle group pulling the *hyoid bone* and *larynx* upward and downward: the *laryngeal elevators,* which are the suprahyoid and longitudinal muscles of the pharynx, and the *laryngeal depressors*, corresponding to the infrahyoid muscles (**see also Anterior Neck Region**).
- View the **cricothyroid muscle**, which you should **differentiate from the remaining intrinsic muscles**, because it is the only muscle of the larynx innervated by the *superior laryngeal nerve (external branch)*. Discuss how this muscle controls the *tension of the vocal cords*, and why the *height of the voice* is different in adult males and females (larger thyroid cartilage or Adam's apple in males).

- Find the **other intrinsic laryngeal muscles**, which are all supplied by the *inferior laryngeal nerve*:

The intrinsic muscles of the larynx that **close the vestibular opening** during swallowing are the aryepiglottic, thyroepiglottic and thyroarytenoid muscles.

The only *abductors* of vocal folds that **open the vocal folds** are the *posterior cricoarytenoid muscles (rt. and lt.)*.

When the vocal folds are in an open position, the *lateral cricoarytenoid muscles* **close (adduct)** the *intermembranous part* of the vocal cords, and the *transverse and oblique arytenoid muscles* close the *intercartilaginous part* of vocal cords.

In addition to the *cricothyroid muscle* mentioned above, the *vocalis muscle* also controls the **tension of vocal folds** by *shortening (relaxing)* them.

• **Blood supply of the larynx**

- View the **superior thyroid artery** from the external carotid artery, and the **inferior thyroid artery** arising from the thyrocervical trunk (branch of subclavian artery). The two arteries give rise to the *superior* and *inferior laryngeal arteries*, respectively.

- Find the paired **superior laryngeal veins** draining into the superior thyroid vein. The *latter veins* eventually drain either directly or indirectly (through the common facial vein) into the *internal jugular vein*.

- Find the paired **inferior laryngeal veins**, which drain often only into the (unpaired) **left inferior thyroid vein**. The latter vein eventually drains into the *left brachiocephalic vein*.

Coniotomy (laryngotomy) is a cut made through the *cricothyroid membrane* (including median cricothyroid ligament) *between the thyroid and cricoid cartilages* in an **acute life-threatening emergency**, e.g. a swelling in the laryngopharynx or upper larynx after a bee-sting.

Endotracheal intubation is a placement of a tube into the trachea to keep the airways open in an emergency or for artificial respiration during surgery. Oral intubation is usually used during brief surgical procedures, in which no complications are expected. For longer intubations (e.g. in an intensive care unit), a nasal intubation or a tracheotomy are required.

Tracheotomy (or tracheostomy) is a surgical opening of the *trachea* approximately between the 4th-5th tracheal cartilages under anaesthesia. After incising the *skin with the subcutaneous tissue* and the *platysma*, the *strap muscles (four infrahyoid muscles)* are separated in the midline. In a next step, a cut is made between the tracheal cartilages, and a respiratory tube is inserted into the trachea, which is connected to a respiratory apparatus until the patient starts to breath spontaneously.

10.3 BACKGROUND INFORMATION

- **Breathing**

The larynx is required for **air passage** from the pharynx to trachea, and **prevents food from entering** into the trachea by closing the laryngeal lumen (passive closure of epiglottis - see below).

During respiration the *lumen of the larynx* is open, because the *epiglottis* is in an upright position, and the *vocal folds* are open. During **quiet respiration or whispering**, only the *intercartilaginous part* of the vocal folds is open. During more **intense breathing** both the *intercartilaginous and intermembranous parts* of the vocal folds are open, and the wideness of the opening depends on the intensity of breathing (e.g. widely opened during forced respiration).

A **unilateral damage** to the recurrent laryngeal nerve (e.g. during surgery of the thyroid gland, **see Deep Neck Region**) will cause hoarseness. **Bilateral nerve damage** can result in severe breathing difficulties, and the inability to speak (aphonia).

- **Swallowing**

Swallowing starts, when the food is pressed by the *dorsum of the tongue* against the *hard palate*, and the **gag reflex** is initiated.

In a next step, the nasopharynx is **sealed involuntarily** by the *elevation of the soft palate* and *contraction of the superior constrictor* of the pharynx. This induces an elevation on the posterior nasopharynx called the **Passavant's pad** (or Passavant's ridge or cushion).

Now the **hyoid bone and larynx** are **elevated** by the *suprahyoid muscles* supported by the *laryngeal elevators* (stylopharyngeus and palatopharyngeus muscles).

The *vestibular opening of larynx* is closed passively, because the *mass of tongue* presses the epiglottis downward at its root, when the hyoid bone and larynx are elevated. Thus, the **passive closure of the larynx** results from the action of the suprahyoid muscles and laryngeal elevators as described above.

The **peristaltic movements** of the *pharyngeal constrictors* transport the bolus downward, and the bolus enters the *oesophagus*.

The **gag reflex** (*pharyngeal reflex*) is the contraction of pharyngeal and palatal muscles induced by objects touching the soft palate. It helps us to avoid choking by preventing objects from entering the throat (except food). The reflex has an *afferent limb* relaying sensory information through the glossopharyngeal nerve (CN. IX), and an *efferent limb* for motor innervation by the glossopharyngeal (CN. IX), vagus (CN. X), and cranial root of the accessory nerves (CN.XI), which all have their origin in the *nucleus ambiguus* in the brainstem.

- **Speech**

During **speech** we distinguish phonation from articulation.

For **phonation** the *larynx* is required. Phonation is the regulation of the **height of the voice** by modification of the tension of the vocal cords. During phonation *both parts of the vocal folds* are open (intercartilaginous and intermembranous parts), but the opening of the *intermembranous part* is *very narrow*.

Articulation is the formation of different sounds (vocals and consonants) by movements of the lips, the tongue, palate and pharynx. The resonance of the voice is further increased by the paranasal air sinuses filled with air. Therefore, we are still able to whisper in the absence of phonation (no voice).

A *weakness* or *incoordination of muscles* required for speech and swallowing will result in a **dysarthria** and **dysphagia**, respectively. Dysarthria and dysphagia can be caused by *peripheral* (e.g. facial nerve palsy) or *central lesion*s [e.g. motor neuron disorder or bulbar palsy after stroke, which can affect the cranial nerve nuclei (lower motor neuron disease) or motor cortex/corticonuclear tracts (upper motor neuron disease)].

A *mechanical obstruction* of the oesophagus can also lead to *dysphagia*, e.g. a *pharyngeal pouch*, which is a pathological hernia of the pharyngeal mucosa through the muscles of the pharynx at the *Killian's triangle* (triangular area between the inferior pharyngeal constrictor and cricopharyngeus muscles). It can displace the oesophagus laterally when it enlarges. It can further cause respiratory problems if an *aspiration* of pouch contents occurs (entry into larynx and lower air ways).

- **Autonomic nervous system**

Cell Bodies of Visceral Motor Neurons in the **Sympathetic System***:*

Preganglionic neurones	**Thoracolumbar region** of the spinal cord (intermediolateral nucleus or lateral gray horns of spinal cord segments, from T1 to L2 / 3)
Preganglionic fibres	**Ventral root** of spinal nerve, **white ramus communicans** of the spinal nerve, ramus interganglionares
Postganglionic neurones	1) **Paravertebral ganglia** (sympathetic chain or trunk consisting of 3 cervical ganglia, 11 thoracic ganglia, 4 lumbar ganglia, 4 sacral ganglia, and 1 ganglion impar) 2) **Prevertebral ganglia** (e.g. celiac ganglion)
Postganglionic fibres	Reach target organs in two ways: 1) join the spinal nerve as **gray ramus communicans** 2) course in the **walls of vessels**, e.g. internal plexus of carotid artery

Cell Bodies of Visceral motor Neurons in the **Parasympathetic System***:*

Preganglionic neurones	Cell bodies in **two separate regions of CNS** 1) **nuclei** of cranial nerves CN. III, CN. VII, CN. IX, CN. X 2) **lateral gray horns** of spinal cord segments **S2-4**
Preganglionic fibres	The preganglionic parasympathetic fibres may have **very tortuous** courses: 1) for preganglionic parasympathetic fibres in **cranial nerves** (see **Practical Session** on **Reconstruction of Course of Cranial nerves**). 2) preganglionic parasympathetic fibres from **sacral segments** leave the spinal cord within the *ventral roots* of spinal nerves, branch off from the *anterior ramus* of spinal nerves, and course as *pelvic splanchnic nerves* until they reach the *autonomic pelvic plexus*, where they mix up with pre- and postganglionic sympathetic fibres. They usually reach their targets in the **walls of vessels** together with postganglionic sympathetic fibres (e.g. vesicular plexus)
Postganglionic neurones	Again there are some differences in the localisation of cell bodies in the **cranial and caudal divisions** of the parasympathetic system: 1) cell bodies in **special ganglia** (e.g. ciliary ganglion; pterygopalatine ganglion; submandibular ganglion; otic ganglion) 2) cell bodies in the **target organs themselves** or in **their vicinity** (e.g. ganglion cells in the submucosa of the larynx for the innervation of laryngeal glands; ganglia embedded in cardiac plexus; intramural ganglia in the wall of oesophagus, stomach or intestine; pelvic ganglion)
Postganglionic fibres	Reach target organs in two ways: 1) join **other cranial nerves** (e.g. postganglionic fibres of chorda tympani nerve coursing back from the submandibular ganglion to the lingual nerve, and reaching the submandibular, sublingual, and lingual glands in the anterior 2/3 rd of the tongue) 2) mostly **axons** of local intramural ganglionic neurons **in the target areas** (e.g. subepicardial plexus of the heart, intramural ganglia of intestine). Often these are **not specific parasympathetic neurons** (e.g. intramural ganglionic neurons of the intestine)

11. ORBIT

11.1 DISSECTIONS

- **Opening of the orbit**
- **Remove the brain** if not done before.
- Remove the **frontal bone** contributing to the *roof of the orbit* up to the *lesser wing of the sphenoid bone* and the *superior orbital fissure*. Chisel about 1 cm of the bone above the **superior orbital fissure** and remove it. Also remove a **stripe of 0.5 mm** from the *lateral part of the* **ethmoid bone**.
- Now you will see the **periorbital membrane** (dense connective tissue and extension of dura mater into orbit) and the **mucosa** covering the ethmoidal cells (paranasal air sinuses).
- Open the periorbital membrane crosswise and reflect its four wings laterally.

- **Contents of the orbit**
- Gently remove the *adipose tissue* (corpus adiposum orbitae) with a **blunt tweezers** (***not scalpel***) to mobilise the nerves, vessels and muscles!
- Find the **ophthalmic nerve** *(CN. V_1)* entering the orbit through the superior orbital fissure and dividing into the *frontal, nasociliary* and *lacrimal nerves*.

  Reveal the **frontal nerve** coursing in the middle with the *supraorbital* and *supratrochlear branches*.

  Reveal the **nasociliary nerve** coursing medially with its *anterior* and *posterior ethmoidal branches*, and the *long* and *short ciliary branches*.

  Reveal the **lacrimal nerve** coursing laterally to reach the lacrimal gland.
- Find the **levator palpaebrae superioris** and **superior rectus muscles** and the *superior division* of the *oculomotor nerve (CN. III)* innervating these muscles. Dissect the nerve coursing just beneath the superior rectus muscle.
- Carefully dissect the **ciliary ganglion** below the superior rectus muscle embedded in a *network of nerve fibres* originating from the *oculomotor nerve* and joining branches of the *nasociliary nerve* (long and short ciliary branches).
- Find the **abducens nerve** coursing laterally until it reaches the **lateral rectus muscle** and clean up its branches entering the muscle to innervate it.
- Find the **trochlear nerve** coursing medially and innervating the *superior oblique muscle*.
- Finally, find the **remaining orbital muscles** (*inferior rectus muscle, medial rectus muscle* and *inferior oblique muscle*) innervated by the *inferior division* of the *oculomotor nerve*.
- View the ophthalmic artery (branch of internal carotid) entering the orbit together with the optic nerve through the optic canal, and the sup. & inf. ophthalmic veins.

11.2 PROSECTIONS AND MODELS

- **Eye ball**

Study the **interior of an eye:**

- View the *three layers* of the *eye ball* (*retina*, *choroid* and *sclera* in continuation with the *cornea*).

- Inspect the *iris* separating the *anterior eye chamber* (between the cornea and the iris) from the *posterior eye chamber* (between the iris and the lens).

- Identify the *ora serata*, which is the transition zone between the *optic* (or visual) and *ciliary parts of the retina*.

- View the *zonular fibres* holding the *lens* and the *ciliary muscle*, which controls the length and tension of the zonular fibres.

- Find the *ciliary body* (corona ciliaris), which produces the secretion of the two eye chambers *connected* through the *pupil*. The secretion produced in the posterior eye chamber circulates through the pupil to the anterior eye chamber, where it is resorbed by the *scleral venous sinus*.

- Find *scleral venous sinus* (*Schlemm's canal*) located at the *iridocorneal angle* of the anterior eye chamber.

- **Horner's syndrome**

- Mark all potential sites of a lesion, which can lead to a *Horner's syndrome*, on the **neck of a student in your group** with colours used for face painting.

A **Horner's syndrome** results from an interruption of the sympathetic nerve supply to the eye, and is characterised by the classic **triad** of *ptosis* (dropping upper eyelid), *miosis* (constricted pupil), and *enophthalmus* (the impression that the eye is sunk in). **In addition**, there is a *decrease or loss of hemifacial sweating* (anhidrosis), and *conjunctival injection* (blood shot conjunctiva). In children, Horner's syndrome sometimes leads to a difference in eye color between the two eyes (heterochromia) due to lack of sympathetic stimulation.

Potential causes leading to a Horner's syndrome are damage to the **postganglionic sympathetic plexus** around the *carotid arteries* (e.g. trauma, dissection of arterial wall, aneurysms, surgery) or to the *sympathetic trunk* (e.g. bronchial cancer metastasizing to the *stellate ganglion*, malignancies in the neck).

A damage to **preganglionic fibres** can occur in pathological conditions affecting the *ventral roots of spinal nerves* from the segments *T1 to L2 / 3* (e.g. trauma, polyradiculitis as a results of an infection like borrelliosis, etc.) or the sympathetic trunk (e.g. damage to preganglionic fibres in rami interganglionares).

Please note that an interruption of **central sympathetic nerve fibres** can also cause a Horner's syndrome, e.g. a lesion in the intermediolateral nucleus of the spinal cord or hypothalamus in the brain.

---

12. PTERYGOPALATINE GANGLION, TEMPORAL BONE, NASAL CAVITY & PARANASAL AIR SINUSES

The aim is to dissect the **pterygopalatine ganglion**, reveal the *course of the facial nerve* in the **temporal bone** (with branches of *nervus intermedius*). The *ear* and the *nasal cavity & paranasal air sinuses* will also be studied.

12.1 DISSECTIONS

- **Pterygopalatine ganglion**
- **Remove** a 1-2 cm thick **vertical stripe of the mucosa** of the **nasal cavity** starting from the *posterior border of the middle nasal choncha* downwards. The stripe should remain anterior to the *torus tubarius*, and the *opening* of the *pharyngotympanic (auditory) tube*.
- Mobilise the **mucosa of the palate** starting from the *soft palate* towards the *hard palate* (posterior-anterior direction), and find the **greater palatine nerve** coursing between the mucosa and the hard palate (formed by the horizontal plate of palatine bone and palatine process of maxilla).
- Along the vertical line between the middle nasal choncha and greater palatine nerve carefully chisel the bone to **remove the medial plate** of the *pterygoid process* of the sphenoid bone and the **perpendicular plate** of the *palatine bone*.
- Now you reached the **pterygopalatine fossa** from medially. This will give you an idea, how far the fossa extends medially. Carefully remove the connective tissue around the *pterygopalatine ganglion* with a **blunt tweezers** to mobilise the ganglion, and find the *branches of the maxillary nerve* in the fossa.

- **Course of the facial nerve in the temporal bone**
- **Remove the dura** in the middle cranial cavity above the **petrous part** of the *temporal bone* (also called *petrosal bone*), and find the following **openings**:

  (1) *Hiatus and grove* of the *greater petrosal nerve* (from intermediate division of CN. VII, courses medially),

  (2) *Hiatus and grove* of the *lesser petrosal nerve* (from the tympanic nerve from the CN. IX, courses laterally). The two grooves course from their hiatuses (openings) towards the *foramen lacerum* on their way to the pterygopalatine ganglion and otic ganglion, respectively.

  (3) *Internal acoustic meatus*, where the facial (CN. VII) and vestibulocochlear (CN. VIII) nerves enter the *petrous portion of the temporal bone*.

- Along the **line between the hiatus of the greater petrosal nerve** and the **internal acoustic meatus** carefully **chisel the bone** (not wider than 0.5 - 1 cm). Once you have removed the bone you will be able to **find** the *facial (CN. VII)* and *vestibulocochlear (CN. VIII)* nerves and follow their course until the **geniculate ganglion**.

- Starting at the geniculate ganglion, the *facial nerve* makes a sharp bend and changes its course to a *latero-posterior direction* towards the **stylomastoid foramen**.
- In the **angle** between the **proximal part of the facial nerve** and the **greater petrosal nerve** you will find the *bony and membranous parts of the cochlea*.
- In the **angle** between the **proximal and distal parts of the facial nerve** you will find the bony and membranous parts of the *semicircular canals*.
- Remove the **petrous bone lateral to** the *greater petrosal nerve* and *distal part* of the *facial nerve*, which is the **roof of the tympanic cavity**. This will allow you to see the tympanic cavity with the ossicles called *malleus*, *incus* and *stapes*, as well as the *tympanic membrane* (ear drum).

12.2 PROSECTIONS AND MODELS

- **Bony and membranous labyrinths in the temporal bone**
- Find the *external opening* of the *vestibular aqueduct* in the petrosal part of the temporal bone containing the *endolymphatic duct and sac* (superior skull base).
- Turn the skull and search for the *external opening* of the *cochlear canaliculus and aqueduct* at the inferior aspect of the skull base (perilymphatic space connected to subarachnoid space), which is localised between the *openings* of the *carotid canal* and *jugular foramen* just behind the *tympanic canaliculus*.

- **External nose and nasal cavity**
- Recapitulate the bony and cartilaginous elements forming the *external nose*, the borders of the *nasal cavity* including the *nasal septum*. Also examine the nasal *conchae*, *meatuses* and *turbinates*, and remember that the *nasolacrimal duct* opens into the inferior meatus of the nose (**see Skull-II Practical**).
- Delineate the part of the nasal cavity containing the **olfactory epithelium** (or mucosa) required for the **sensation of smell** on the *superior nasal concha* and *upper third of nasal septum* (see Neuroanatomy books for further details).
- Note that the **rest of the nasal cavity** is covered with **respiratory epithelium** as the nasal cavity is the upper portion of the respiratory tract (see **Histology** books).
- View the *lateral and septal arteries* in the **anterior and posterior halves** of the nasal cavity:

  1) Anterior half: *anterolateral and septal arteries* originating from the *ant.* and *post. ethmoidal arteries* (from ophthalmic artery from *internal carotid* artery – they course from the orbit via the ethmoid sinuses and cribriform plate to the nasal cavity).

  2) Posterior half: *posterolateral and septal arteries* originating from *sphenopalatine artery* (from maxillary artery from *external carotid* artery – they course from pterygopalatine fossa through sphenopalatine foramen to the nasal cavity).

- View the **nerve supply to the external nose** (*nasal branches* of the *infraorbital* and *anterior superior alveolar nerves*), and to the **nasal cavity** (*anterior* and *posterior ethmoidal nerves, short sphenopalatine nerves, long sphenopalatine nerve*, and *internal nasal branch* of the *anterior superior alveolar nerve*).

Epistaxis is nosebleed draining out through the nostrils and/or through the choanae into the stomach. The most frequent site of epistaxis is localised in the *anterior portion* of the *nasal septum*, especially in the *Kieselbach's area* (or Little's area), where several converging arteries form anastomoses. Posterior epistaxis is less common, but usually more severe.

Rhinorrhea is a drippy nose, when the nasal mucosa produces large amounts of secretion due to a rhinitis (nose infection). Rhinorrhea should be differentiated from **liquorrhea** (or cerebrospinal fluid rhinorrhea) if cerebrospinal fluid drops out of the nose, because the dura and arachnoid mater are damaged in the anterior cranial cavity, which happens most frequently at the *cribriform lamina.*

- **Paranasal air sinuses**
- Localise the **boundaries of the maxillary air sinus** formed by *different portions* of the *maxillary bone*. The **roof** of the maxillary sinus is formed by a thin plate separating the sinus from the orbit. Its **floor** extends into the alveolar bone of the maxilla, into which the roots of upper teeth can protrude (1st and 2nd molars, as well as variably the 3rd molar, premolars & canines). The **medial wall** separates the maxillary sinus from the nasal cavity, and the **lateral wall** extends to the zygomatic process of the maxilla.
- View the shape and extension of the **frontal, ant. & post. ethmoidal** and **sphenoidal air sinuses**.
- Inspect the openings of the air sinuses into the nasal cavity:

  The frontal sinus, maxillary sinus and anterior ethmoidal sinuses drain into the **middle nasal meatus**: the *frontal sinus* into hiatus semilunaris via the infundibulum, the *maxillary sinus* through *own ostium* medial to the hiatus semilunaris, and the *anterior ethmoidal sinuses* (incl. *bulla ethmoidalis*) either directly into middle nasal meatus or indirectly through the frontal infundibulum at the hiatus semilunaris.

  The *posterior ethmoidal sinuses* drain directly into the **superior meatus of nose**.

  The *sphenoid sinus* drains into the **sphenoethmoidal recess** at anterior wall of sphenoid sinus.

- View the **nerve and blood supply** of the paranasal air sinuses in the diagram below. Also note that the *superior alveolar* and *superior pharyngeal arteries* both originate from the *maxillary artery*, which is a branch of the *external carotid artery.*

The **maxillary sinus** has a higher risk of becoming infected as compared to other paranasal air sinuses, called *sinusitis* (infection of an air sinus), because (i) the ostium draining the secretion of the sinus into the middle nasal meatus is localised much higher than the floor of the sinus, and a *pulpitis of upper teeth* (infection at the root of a tooth) can easily penetrate the maxillary sinus.

Innervation of Paranasal Air Sinuses
mainly by Branches of Trigeminal Nerve

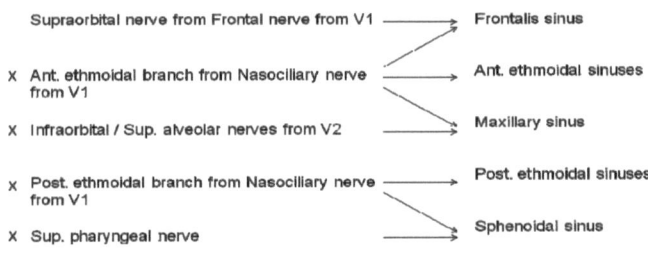

x: *accompanying blood vessels with the same names (e.g. ant. ethmoidal artery)*

- **Outer and middle ear**

- View the **nerve and blood supply** of the paranasal air sinuses in the diagram below. Also note that the *superior alveolar* and *superior pharyngeal arteries* both originate from the *maxillary artery*, which is a branch of the *external carotid artery*.

- Delineate the components of the **external ear** (visible flap of tissue or ear called *auricle* or pinna, and *external auditory meatus*), **middle ear** (*tympanic cavity*, which is connected to the *pharyngotympanic tube* also called *Eustachian tube* or *auditory tube*) and **inner ear** (*bony labyrinth* and *membranous labyrinth*).

- View the **external auditory meatus** with its *cartilaginous portion* connected to the auricle and its *bony parts*. The bony part of the external auditory meatus is formed by the squamous (superiorly), and tympanic parts (everywhere else) of the temporal bone.

- View the **lateral** (*bony canal*) **and medial borders** (*cartilaginous and membranous*) of the **pharyngotympanic (auditory) tube** coursing from the *nasopharynx* to the *tympanic cavity*.

- Describe the **boundaries of** and **major structures in** the **middle ear cavity**: the **roof** (tegmen tympani from petrous part of temporal bone), **medial wall** (inner ear), **lateral wall** (tympanic membrane), **anterior wall** (opening of pharyngotympanic tube and tendon of tensor tympani muscle), **posterior wall** (opening of mastoid antrum or aditus, canal of facial nerve and the pyramid formed by the stapedius muscle), and **floor** (thin bony segment above jugular bulb).

- Describe/name the **ossicles** in middle ear cavity (malleus, incus and stapes), and the function of the **tensor tympani** and **stapedius muscles**.

The *external auditory meatus* and *tympanic membrane* (ear drum) receive their **sensory innervation** mainly from the *auricular branch of the auriculotemporal nerve*. The *auricular branch of the vagus nerve* coursing from the superior vagal ganglion to the external acoustic meatus (through the mastoid canaliculus and tympanomastoid fissure) only innervates *a small area* at the posterior and inferior part of the meatus. Still dropping a cold solution into the ear can induce *bradycardia* resulting from an activation of a **vago-vagal reflex** (induced by stimulation of vagal afferents, e.g. also after endotracheal intubation).

Otitis media is an acute (mostly secretary) or chronic infection of the **middle ear cavity**, which can be very painful. It often results from a disturbed air circulation in the middle ear, when the pharyngeal entrance of the pharyngotympanic (auditory) tube is blocked by a swelling of the mucosa or an enlargement of tonsils (pharyngeal and/or tubar tonsils). Otitis media is **relevant to dentistry**, because *temporomandibular joint (TMJ) disorders* or *infections of the parotid gland* can result in pain symptoms **referred to the ear**. Furthermore, otitis media can damage structures in the tympanic cavity including the **chorda tympani nerve** and the adjacent inner ear. It can also *spread* to the **mastoid cells** (pneumatic bone) and damage the **facial nerve** there, lead to a **subperiosteal abscess** (can penetrate the *TMJ* and region behind the *tendon of the sternocleidomastoid muscle*) or infiltrate the *tegmen tympani* causing an **intracranial abscess** or **sigmoid sinus thrombosis**. One common complication of chronic otitis media is *cholesteatoma* (benign growth of skin into the tympanic cavity or mastoid cells following a defect of the ear drum).

Meniere's disease is a disorder of the **inner ear** affecting balance & hearing associated with vertigo, dizziness, tinnitus & loss of hearing. *Vertigo* is the abnormal sensation of movements like spinning or whirling associated with dizziness, faintness or unsteadiness. *Tinnitus* is the perception of sounds in form of ringing, whining, buzzing or clicking in the ear despite the lack of any comparable sounds in the environment. Note that similar symptoms also occur in **TMJ disorders**.

- **Inner ear**

The inner ear is composed of the *bony* and *membranous labyrinths*, the latter residing within the bony labyrinth and surrounded by *perilymph*. The membranous labyrinth is a closed tubular system filled with *endolymph*.
- The *cochlea* required for hearing has a membranous labyrinth with the *organ of Corti* and a bony labyrinth divided into the *scala tympani & vestibuli*, both filled with perilymph. The organ of Corti contains *hair cells* that reside on the *basilar membrane* and reach to the *tectorial membrane* (gel-like structure). The basilar membrane vibrates in a frequency-specific manner if activated by sound waves. The cochlea is connected to the middle ear through the *oval* (at the *vestibule*) & *round windows* (at the *scala tympani*) to balance out the vibration pressure.
- The *semicircular canals* (three half-circular tubes running in three different planes), *saccule* and *utricle* belong to vestibular system important for balance.
- Cochlear neurons are located in the **spiral** and vestibular neurons in the **vestibular ganglion** (their axons form the vestibulocochlear nerve, CN. VIII).

13. RECONSTRUCTION OF THE COURSE OF CRANIAL NERVES III, V1-3, VII AND IX

We will **reconstruct** the pathway of the trigeminal branches carrying autonomic fibres to the target organs with the **aid of threads and sellotape**. Threads in different **colours** will be used to distinguish the branches of individual nerves.

Use a different plastic skull for each reconstruction. Compare the skulls with **real skulls**, e.g. to find the pterygoid canal or to view the foramen lacerum.

13.1 RECONSTRUCTION OF NERVES

• **Oculomotor nerve (CN. III) - Autonomic fibres to orbit**

1) Take <u>two red</u> threads and <u>one orange</u> thread. Pull all three threads through the carotid canal, and fix them at the carotid canal with sellotape. One red thread is the **internal carotid artery** and the other one is the **ophthalmic artery**. The orange thread corresponds to **postganglionic sympathetic fibres** (carotid plexus).

2) Pull one red thread through the *optic canal* (*ophthalmic artery*) and the orange thread through the *superior orbital fissure* (*postganglionic sympathetic fibres*).

3) Now, take <u>one blue</u> and <u>one green</u> thread. Using sellotape fix them on the clivus and lateral to the sella turcica (position of cavernous sinus). Next pull the tips of the two threads through the *superior orbital fissure*. The blue thread is the **motor division of the oculomotor nerve** (CN. III), and the green thread the **preganglionic parasympathetic division of the oculomotor nerve**.

4) Make a knot between the orange and green threads in the orbit to mark the **ciliary ganglion**, at which the preganglionic parasympathetic fibres form synapses with postganglionic neurones. At this point the *postganglionic sympathetic fibres* also join the *parasympathetic ones*.

(5) Did you notice what is missing?! The autonomic fibres should reach the eye ball together with a **sensory branch of the trigeminal nerve** like other autonomic fibres in the head and neck. These trigeminal branches in the orbit are the **short and long ciliary nerves** (from *nasociliary nerve* from *ophthalmic nerve*):

Take <u>three yellow</u> threads, all of which correspond to the first division of the trigeminal nerve, the **ophthalmic nerve** (CN. V$_1$). Fix all three yellow threads lateral to the sella turcica (position of cavernous sinus) with sellotape, and pull them through the *superior orbital fissure*.

(6) Bring the orange and green threads (their portions after the knot) as well as one of the yellow threads together, and fix them on the posterior surface of a self-made *eye ball* out of paper. When you place your eye ball in the orbit, you will have completed the reconstruction of the terminal portion of **postganglionic parasympathetic** and **postganglionic sympathetic fibres** coursing together with the *short and long ciliary nerves*. The latter nerve carries *sensory fibres to the eye ball* for its **sensory innervation** (e.g. for the corneal reflex).

- **Greater petrosal nerve from facial nerve (CN. VII) - Autonomic fibres to nasal, palatal and pharyngeal mucosa and lacrimal gland**

(1) Take <u>one green</u> thread and fix it on the petrous bone just above the *internal acoustic meatus*. This should mark the projection of the **greater petrosal nerve** onto the surface of the petrous bone at its *entrance* into the temporal bone (autonomic division of the facial nerve).

(2) Place the green thread so that it courses first in *anterolateral* direction. Then make it bend towards *anteromedially* (at putative geniculate ganglion, where the nerve leaves the facial nerve without synapsing). Finally, fix the green thread at the *hiatus* of the *greater petrosal nerve* using sellotape. Now you have marked the position, at which the greater petrosal nerve *exits* the temporal bone.

(4) Take <u>one red</u> thread **(carotid artery)** and <u>one orange</u> thread (**postganglionic sympathetic fibres** in the *carotid plexus*), and pull them together through the carotid canal. Bring the tip of the green thread coming out of the *hiatus* of the greater petrosal nerve and the orange thread intracranially together. Now, we have formed the **nerve of the pterygoid canal** (*Vidian nerve* containing *postganglionic sympathetic fibres* from *deep petrosal nerve* and *preganglionic parasympathetic fibres* from the *greater petrosal nerve*).

(5) Move "your *nerve of the pterygoid canal*" (green and orange threads) toward the foramen lacerum, and fix it with a sellotape within the foramen. Cut the rest of the tip off, so that the nerve does not come out of the foramen lacerum on the inferior skull base. Now we have marked the entrance of the respective nerve to the *pterygoid canal*.

(6) The pterygoid canal is usually missing in plastic skulls. Therefore, take <u>four new green</u> and <u>four new orange</u> threads, and make a knot with them very close to the common tip of all threads. Fix the short end and the knot at the *pterygopalatine fossa* using sellotape. Now you have marked the *exit* of the "*nerve of the pterygoid canal*" and the **pterygopalatine ganglion**, respectively, which are both localised in the pterygopalatine fossa. Please note that the fossa is usually much flatter in plastic skulls than in real ones.

(7) Take <u>four yellow</u> threads corresponding to branches of the **maxillary nerve** (CN. V_2), and starting at the *middle cranial fossa* pull them through the *foramen rotundum*, which has its exit also in the *pterygopalatine fossa*. (If this is not the case *in plastic skulls*, you will have to fix <u>four new yellow</u> threads at the entrance and exit points of the foramen as described for the Vidian nerve, see above).

(8) Bring one thread of each colour together (free long ends of green and orange threads after the knot). You have now four potential *branches of the maxillary nerve* carrying **sensory** and **postganglionic autonomic fibres** *(parasympathetic and sympathetic)* to different regions supplied by the maxillary nerve.

(a) Bring one thread of each colour corresponding to the **infraorbital nerve** through the inferior orbital fissure into the orbit, and let it enter and exit the infraorbital foramen. Discuss the regions of the *face and paranasal air sinuses* (including mucosal glands) innervated by the infraorbital nerve.

(b) Reconstruct the course of the **short sphenopalatine nerves** (from pterygopalatine fossa through sphenopalatine foramen to nasal cavity), the **greater palatine nerve** (from pterygopalatine fossa through greater palatine foramen to hard palate), and the **zygomatic nerve** (from infraorbital fissure through orbit to the face). They innervate the *mucosa and glands* of the *posterior nasal cavity* and *hard palate*, and the *skin of the face* and the *lacrimal gland* (anastomosis with lacrimal nerve), respectively.

- **Chorda tympani nerve from facial nerve (CN. VII) - Autonomic fibres to submandibular & sublingual glands, and sensation of taste**

(1) Take <u>two green</u> threads and <u>one blue</u> thread, and fix them on the petrous bone just above the *internal acoustic meatus* to mark the *entrance* of the **chorda tympani nerve** (green) and **motor division of the facial nerve** (blue) into the meatus projected onto the surface of the petrous bone. The chorda tympani nerve carrying fibres for autonomic innervation and the sensation of taste is part of the *nervus intermedius* like the greater petrosal nerve (latter carries autonomic fibres only). Hence, the nervus intermedius includes both the greater petrosal nerve and chorda tympani, and is part of the whole (mixed) facial nerve.

(2) Place the two green threads and the blue thread so that they course in an *antero-lateral direction* toward the *hiatus* of the *greater petrosal nerve*. Make a knot into one of the green threads only, which should lie *exactly on the hiatus*. Fix the green knot, the second green thread without a knot, and the blue thread around the region of the hiatus of the greater petrosal nerve using sellotape. Now you have marked the position of the **geniculate ganglion**, where the **gustatory ganglionic neurons** of the *chorda tympani nerve* are localised (taste sensation to the tongue). The *autonomic fibres* of the chorda tympani nerve *pass through* this ganglion *without synapsing here*!

(3) At "our geniculate ganglion" (green knot around hiatus of the greater petrosal nerve) *bend* our two green threads and one blue thread *sharply* into a posterolateral direction by moving the terminal portions of the threads toward the *stylomastoid foramen*. Until this point the chorda tympani nerve has the *same course* in the temporal bone like the *motor division* of the *facial nerve*.

(4) Of course, we only marked the projection of the chorda tympani nerve onto the outer surface of the temporal bone. In reality, the nerve courses within the bone. Nevertheless, we can imitate the last peculiarity in the intracranial course of the chorda tympani nerve now by fixing our two green threads and blue thread above the stylomastoid foramen. This is the point, where the chorda tympani nerve *leaves* the *motor division* of the *facial nerve* and starts its short journey on its own (until it joins the lingual nerve). Cut the rest of the blue thread above the stylomastoid foramen to indicate that the motor division of the facial nerve leaves the skull through the *stylomastoid foramen*.

(5) To finalise the reconstruction of the course of the chorda tympani nerve within the temporal bone, we have to move the tips of our two green threads anteriorly, and fix them again using sellotape just above the *petrotympanic fissure*. Cut the

rest of the green threads above the petrotympanic fissure. This shall remind us that the chorda tympani nerve courses in the *tympanic cavity* anteriorly between the *ossicles malleus and incus*, and exits the skull at the petrotympanic fissure.

(6) Now take underline four green threads and fix them at the *petrotympanic fissure* outside of the skull using sellotape. This will be the portion of the chorda tympani nerve leaving the skull, and coursing extracranially.

(7) Take four yellow threads and pull them through the *foramen ovale* corresponding to the **mandibular nerve** (CN. V_3).

(8) Bring three of the yellow threads (*lingual nerve*) together with the four green threads (1 thread for **gustatory** and 3 threads for **preganglionic parasympathetic fibres** of the *chorda tympani nerve*). All seven threads should course together until they reach the *submandibular triangle*.

(9) At the submandibular triangle make a knot to mimic the **submandibular ganglion** using 3 green threads (*preganglionic parasympathetic fibres* from the *chorda tympani nerve*). After the "ganglion" let the lingual nerve (3 yellow threads) course together with **postganglionic parasympathetic fibres** of the chorda tympani nerve (3 green threads coming back from the knot), and the **afferent taste fibres** running in the chorda tympani nerve (1 extra green thread).

(10) Take three orange threads (postganglionic sympathetic fibres).

(a) Fix one green (postganglionic parasympathetic fibres), one orange (postganglionic sympathetic fibres) and one yellow thread (branch of lingual nerve) to a self-made *submandibular gland* (paper ball) for its **postganglionic parasympathetic, postganglionic sympathetic** and **sensory innervation**.

(b) Take two green threads (one coming from the submandibular ganglion, and one passing by without knot), one orange, and one yellow thread to the *anterior 2/3^{rds} of the tongue* in the oral cavity (**postganglionic parasympathetic, gustatory, sympathetic** and **sensory innervation, respectively**).

(c) One remaining thread of each colour is for the innervation of the *sublingual gland* (innervation like submandibular gland).

P.S. Postganglionic sympathetic fibres innervating the submandibular and sublingual glands originate from the external carotid artery and reach their targets in the **walls of vessels** (facial and/or lingual artery).

- **Lesser petrosal nerve (CN. IX) – Autonomic supply of the parotid gland**

(1) Take two green threads (*gustatory* and *preganglionic parasympathetic fibres*), and one yellow and two blue threads (*sensory* and/or *motor fibres*) for the **glossopharyngeal nerve**. Make two knots into **one of the green threads only** to mark the **superior ganglion** and **inferior ganglion** of the glossopharyngeal nerve (sensory and gustatory ganglionic neurones).

(2) Fix all five threads in the *intracranial cavity* above the *jugular foramen* using sellotape, and pull them through the jugular foramen toward extracranially. From

the two knots on one green thread ("our ganglions"), one should be localised just above and the other just below jugular foramen.

(3) Fix one yellow and one blue thread as well as the green thread with the two knots together using sellotape. This is the **main branch of the glossopharyngeal nerve** *coursing downward* along with the *stylopharyngeus* muscle (sensory, motor and gustatory innervation of the pharynx, palate, posterior 1/3rd of the tongue).

(4) Bring the other green thread (no knot) and blue thread together. Now, you have reconstructed the **tympanic nerve** containing *preganglionic parasympathetic* and *sensory fibres*. Fix them together at the entrance of the *tympanic canaliculus* to mark the point, where the nerve **re**-enters the temporal bone and heads toward the middle ear.

(5) Find the *hiatus* and *groove* of the *lesser petrosal nerve*, and fix <u>a new green</u> thread *at the hiatus*. This thread corresponds to the terminal branch of the tympanic nerve, called the **lesser petrosal nerve** (*preganglionic parasympathetic fibres*) leaving the temporal bone at the hiatus. The sensory fibres terminate in the middle ear, where they innervate the tympanic air cavity (*tympanic plexus*).

(6) Move "your *lesser petrosal nerve*" (green thread) toward the *foramen lacerum*, pull it through the foramen lacerum toward extracranially, mark the thread with a permanent marker 0.5 cm below the foramen, and make a knot at the marked point (*otic ganglion*). At this stage, you should also fix the portion of the thread coming from the hiatus of the lesser petrosal nerve at the intracranial entrance of the foramen lacerum using sellotape. The knot corresponding to the **otic ganglion** should now lie outside of the skull, and just next to the *foramen ovale*.

(7) Take <u>three new yellow</u> threads corresponding to the **mandibular nerve** (CN. V$_3$), and pull them from intracranial to extracranial through the *foramen ovale*.

(8) Take two of the yellow threads corresponding to the **auriculotemporal nerve**, and join them with the portion of the green thread below your "otic ganglion" (below the green knot). The fibres after the knot correspond to *postganglionic parasympathetic fibres* of the lesser petrosal nerve.

(9) Fix the two yellow threads and the green thread together with sellotape, before you move them together laterally. When you reach the area anterior to the external acoustic meatus, separate the one of the yellow threads. This yellow thread (**main branch of the auriculotemporal nerve**) should make a *sharp bend* here, and *ascend* anteriorly to the external acoustic meatus. Fix this yellow thread with sellotape at the bending point and the temple.

(11) Take one end of a blue thread (**motor portion of the facial nerve** innervating *muscles of facial expression*), and fix it at the *stylomastoid foramen* to mark the exit of the nerve out of the skull.

(12) Take the other end of the blue thread (**motor fibres** *from facial nerve*) to the area anterior to the external acoustic meatus, and bring it together with the green thread (**postganglionic parasympathetic fibres** *from glossopharyngeal nerve*), <u>one new orange</u> thread (**postganglionic sympathetic fibres**), and the remaining yellow thread (**sensory fibres** *from auriculotemporal nerve*). The *motor portion*

of the facial nerve forms a plexus within the parotid gland (**parotid plexus**) together with *autonomic* and *sensory fibres*: the postganglionic parasympathetic fibres originating from the *lesser petrosal nerve* (from glossopharyngeal nerve) and sensory fibres originating from the auriculotemporal nerve (the latter mainly to the capsule). The **postganglionic sympathetic innervation** reaches the **submandibular ganglion** via **branches of the external carotid artery** (mainly from superficial temporal artery).

13.2 RECAPITULATE AT HOME

• Learn about types, location, function, blood supply, and innervation of the **three major salivary glands** (sensory, parasympathetic and sympathetic secretomotor).

• Find the **surface markings** of the parotid, submandibular and sublingual glands, and palpate them on yourself.

• Please note that not only the three major salivary glands, but also the **other salivary glands** having their openings in the oral cavity (including the lingual and palatine glands) as well as the **pharyngeal** and **laryngeal glands** all receive an *autonomic innervation*. **For each of these locations**, identify the trigeminal division (and its end branches) or other cranial nerve (e.g. vagus nerve for the larynx) supplying the sensory innervation. Finally, **name the respective autonomic ganglion**, from where the autonomic fibres are carried to the end organs (e.g. pterygopalatine ganglion for the palatine glands, and intramural ganglion of vagus nerve for laryngeal glands).

• Learn about the opposing effects of the sympathetic and parasympathetic systems. Please note that *preganglionic* neurons use *acetylcholine* as neurotransmitter, whereas *postganglionic parasympathetic* neurons use *acetylcholine*, and *postganglionic sympathetic neurons* use *noradrenalin*.

Sympathetic Stimulation	Parasympathetic Stimulation
"skeletal muscle activity and stress"	*"rest and digestion"*
- salivation ↓	- salivation ↑
- diversion of blood from gut & skin to skeletal muscles	- glandular activity in gut ↑
- pupillary dilatation	- pupillary constriction
- sweating ↑	- no effect on sweat glands ↔
- heart rate, blood pressure↑	- heart rate, blood pressure ↓
- bronchodilatation	- bronchoconstriction, -secretion
- piloerection	- no piloerection
- peristalsis ↓	- peristalsis ↑
- sphincter contraction (bladder)	- bladder (detrusor) contraction, micturition
- tocolysis (uterine relaxation)	- uterine contraction
- erectile tissue function ↓	- erectile tissue function ↑

14. BODY WALL

The body wall protects our inner organs by covering the thoracic and abdominal cavities, and allows different types of movements.

The body wall is formed by various layers. From outward the body wall consists of the *skin* and *subcutaneous* tissue localised just underneath the skin, which is also called *Camper's fatty layer*. Below the subcutaneous tissue, there is straight connective tissue, also called the *Scarpa's fascia or membranous layer*. It covers the next layer consisting of bones, cartilages and muscles. This fascia and the deepest fascia lining the inner body wall are different from the own fascia of individual muscles! The deepest fascia is called *endothoracic fascia* in the **thorax** and *transversalis fascia* in the **abdomen**.

The thoracic and abdominal cavities are separated by the *thoracic diaphragm*, whereas the lower enclosure of the abdominal cavity is formed by the *pelvic* and *urogenital diaphragms*. There is **no diaphragm** separating the neck from the thorax, which facilitates the infiltration of infections or tumours from the neck to the thorax and vice versa. From inside, the thoracic and abdominal cavities are covered by the *parietal pleura* and *parietal peritoneum*, respectively.

In this session we will inspect the **bones, cartilages, fascia and muscles** of the body wall including the **diaphragms**.

14.1 PROSECTIONS AND MODELS

- **Vertebrae**
- Examine the characteristics of *cervical*, *thoracic*, *lumbar*, *sacral* and *coccygeal* **vertebrae** by identifying their body, transverse processes, costal processes (lumbar vertebrae only), laminae, pedicles, spinous processes, articular facets and costal facets.
- Note the **joints** & **ligaments** of the vertebral column (backbone or spine) including those, which form the *intervertebral foramina* around **spinal nerves**. View the *transverse canals* for the **vertebral artery**, and *vertebral canal* of the spinal cord.
- View the *kyphosis* of the thoracic spine (concave anteriorly) and *lordosis* of the cervical & lumbar spine (convex anteriorly). S*coliosis* is an abnormal curvature.
- Inspect the structure of an **intervertebral disc** including the *annulus fibrosus* and *nucleus pulposus*. Describe the **types of movements** of the vertebral column.
- Identify the **spinal cord** terminating at the vertebral level *L1-2 in adults*. Below this level, find the *cauda equina* (dorsal and ventral roots of spinal nerves) and the *filum terminale* (thin extension of spinal cord out of connective tissue). Cerebrospinal fluid can be obtained below L2 by performing a **lumbar puncture** by inserting a needle into the *spinal (or vertebral) canal*.

A *herniated disc* (prolaps of nucleus pulposus out of intervertebral disc) can result from an overload of vertebrae, often caused by flexion in a twisted position. It is most common in *cervical* and *lumbar segments*.

A disc herniation is usually accompanied by other degenerative changes of vertebrae, e.g. a decrease in the *height of the disc, retro- or anterolisthesis of vertebrae* (gliding of vertebrae), thickening of the *ligamentum flavum*, and development of *osteophytes* (degenerative bony extension of vertebrae).

A cervical disc prolaps or retro- or anterolisthesis of cervical vertebrae can lead to *headache, obstruction of the spinal cord* (with paralysis below this segment), and *segmental symptoms* at the level of the lesion by *compressing the spinal nerve* in the intervertebral foramen.

- **Transitional zone between the skull and vertebrae**
- View the **occipital condyles, external occipital protuberance**, and **sup. and inf. nuchal lines**.
- Note the features of the **atlas** and **axis** (first two atypical cervical vertebrae) with the *ant. and post. arches* of the atlas, the *articular facet for the dens*, the *dens of axis* (body of atlas during development) with the facet for the ant. arch of atlas, and the *bifid spinous process, body* and *vertebral arch* of the axis.
- View the *transverse foramen* and *groove* of the *vertebral artery* on the atlas for the course of the **vertebral artery**, which penetrates the *atlanto-occipital membrane* to enter the posterior cranial fossa through the *foramen magnum*.
- Study the *atlanto-occipital* and *atlanto-axial* **joints** with their *ligaments*.

Mechanical dysfunction or hypomobility of the **upper cervical spine** and **transitional zone** can also cause headache. **Disorders of the cranio-cervical transitional zone** (e.g. *traumatic injuries, Arnold-Chiari malformation*) further lead often to neurological symptoms resulting from damage to the lower brainstem, cerebellum and/or upper spinal cord (e.g. tetraparesis).

- **Costae (ribs) and sternum**
- Note characteristics of **ribs** by identifying their *head, neck, tubercle, articular facets, angle* and *subcostal groove* sheltering the **intercostal nerve and vessels**. View the costal cartilages, 9th costal cartilage and costal margin. This will help you to characterise typical and atypical ribs, *costae verae* (true ribs) and *costae spuriae* (false ribs), and *floating ribs* (last two ribs not attached to the sternum).
- Identify the *manubrium, body* and *xiphoid process* of the **sternum**. View the suprasternal notch, sternal angle / angle of Louis.
- Describe the *costovertebral, sternocostal* (formed by the costal cartilages of ribs 1-7 and the sternum) and *costochondral* **joints**.

Cervical ribs forming joints with cervical vertebrae are a **variation**. They can compress vessels like the *subclavian artery* resulting in a transient reduction in the perfusion of the arm.

- **Pelvic girdle**

- View the lt. and rt. **pelvic bones** (*os coxae*) joined at the *pubic symphysis.* Each pelvic bone is composed of an *iliac bone* (*os ilium*), *ishiac bone* (*os ischii*) and *pubic bone* (os pubis). Also view the *iliac crests* and *fossae, anterior superior* and *anterior inferior iliac spines, pubic tubercles* and *ischial tuberosity.*

- Identify the **sacrum, coccyx** (tailbone) and **sacroiliac joints**.

> The **iliac crest** is often used to *harvest bone* for transplants used in bone reconstruction and collect *bone marrow*. Bone marrow can be used for **diagnostic purposes** (e.g. to diagnose blood cancer) or **for transplantation** including autotransplantation, e.g. in **orofacial surgery**.

- **Intrinsic (true) muscles of the body wall**

- **Thoracic cage:**
  Identify the three layers of **intercostal muscles** and the **transversus thoracis muscle**. The *external, internal* and *innermost intercostal muscles* are supplied by branches from the *anterior rami of thoracic spinal nerves* called **intercostal nerves** as well as by **anterior and posterior intercostal vessels** anastomosing at the level of the mid axillary line. Most of these vessels originate from the *internal thoracic artery* and the *descending part of the thoracic aorta*, respectively. The nerve below the 12th rib is called *subcostal nerve*.

- **Abdominal muscles:**
  View the **course of muscle fibres** of the *rectus abdominis, external oblique, internal oblique* and *transversus abdominis muscles*, and compare them with the intercostal muscles. Identify the *umbilicus, linea alba* and *arcuate line* in the posterior wall of the *rectus sheath*.

- **Intrinsic back muscles:**
  View the **superficial** splenius muscle (capitis and cervicis portions), the **intermediate layer** containing the iliocostalis, longissimus and spinalis muscles (erector spinae muscle - in a narrow sense), and **innermost deep muscle group** containing the transversospinalis, semispinalis, multifidus, rotatores and other minor muscles, e.g. the interspinales and intertransversarii. Muscle fibres that insert into the thoracic region are called thoracic, into the cervical region cervicis, and into the skull capitis. All intrinsic muscles of the back can be **summarised according to their course** from their origin to their insertion as *transverso-transversal* (e.g. intertransversarii or iliocostalis), *transverso-spinal* (e.g. semispinales, rotatores), *spino-transversal* (e.g. splenius) and *interspinal* (e.g. spinalis, interspinales). The muscles receive **segmented blood** (e.g. *segmental somatic branches mostly from aorta*) **and nerve supply** from *posterior rami of spinal nerves*.

15. THORAX

In this session, we will study prosections of the **thorax**, and plastic or plastinated models of **thoracic organs**. In addition, the **diaphragm** separating the thorax and abdomen, and structures passing through the diaphragm will be studied.

15.1 PROSECTIONS AND MODELS

- **Mediastinum**

The mediastinum is composed of a group of midline organs and structures separating the rt. and lt. pleural cavities.

- View the **superior mediastinum**, which contains the thoracic inlet from the superior thoracic aperture up to the level, where the pericardial sac around the heart begins. The **inferior mediastinum** is further subdivided into an *anterior mediastinum* occupying the space between the sternum and pericardial sac, *middle mediastinum* containing the pericardial sac, and *posterior mediastinum* containing structures interposed between the pericardial sac and vertebral column.

- **Thymus gland** (lymphoepithelial organ) and **lymph nodes** (paratracheal, tracheobronchial, bronchopulmonary, pulmonary - anterior mediastinal, posterior mediastinal)

- **Trachea and bronchi:** Palpate the *cartilaginous rings* of the trachea and bronchi, view the *bifurcation of the trachea* at the level of the *4th thoracic vertebra* and the *carina* (end of trachea at bifurcation)

- **Heart & its great vessels (blood vessels):** *Pericardial sac* with *heart, aorta* (ascending part, arch, descending part), *brachiocephalic trunk* (only on the right side), *sup. vena cava, inf. vena cava,* and *lt. and rt. brachiocephalic veins, azygous vein, hemiazygous vein, pulmonary trunk* with two pulmonary arteries, *3-5 pulmonary veins.*

- **Phrenic nerves:** Their course in the mediastinal wall and their branches to the mediastinal pleura and pericardium.

- **Rt. and lt. vagus nerves**, and the **recurrent laryngeal nerves** (the rt. recurrent laryngeal nerve looping back behind the rt. subclavian artery and the lt. recurrent laryngeal nerve behind the aortic arch to ascend in the neck)

- **Oesophagus** with **ant. and post. vagal plexus** (ant. vagal plexus from lt. vagus nerve, post. vagal plexus from rt. vagus nerve).

- **Thoracic duct** (biggest lymph vessel) coursing in the posterior mediastinum between the descending thoracic aorta and azygous vein, and heading toward the left venous angle between the left subclavian vein and internal jugular vein.

- **Sympathetic trunk** (also called **sympathetic chain**) during its paravertebral course and the **splanchnic nerves** (greater, lesser, least splanchnic nerves) originating from the trunk.

- **Heart**
- View the **epicardium, myocardium** and **endocardium**. In the pericardial sac find the *transverse pericardial sinus* and *oblique pericardial sinus*.
- Study the **right and left atriums** (incl. auricles) **and ventricles**, the *apex, sup. and inf. vena cava, pulmonary veins, aorta* (ascending part, arch) and *pulmonary trunk*. Inspect the *interatrial septum* (incl. fossa ovalis) and *interventricular septum* (muscular & membranous parts).
- Inspect the **heart skeleton** (connective tissue isolating the atria and ventricles electrically from each other), which is localised at the **level of the four heart valves**, and also surrounds the valves. Study the *pocket* or *semilunar valves* (aortic and pulmonary valves) and the *cuspid valves* (atrio-ventricular or tricuspid and mitral valves) with the *chordae tendineae, papillary muscles*, and *trabeculae carnae*.
- View the openings (above the aortic valve) and course of **coronary arteries**. The *rt. coronary artery* courses in the *coronary sulcus*, and the *post. interventricular branch* (end branch of rt. coronary artery) in *post. interventricular sulcus*. The initial segment of the *left coronary artery* soon divides into the *ant. interventricular branch* coursing in the *ant. interventricular sulcus*, and the *circumflex branch* of left coronary artery coursing in the *lt. coronary sulcus*.
- View the *coronary sinus, terminal groove* (sulcus terminalis), and *christa terminalis*, below which the **sinoatrial node** is localised. Find the position of the **atrioventricular node** at the dorsal wall of the right atrium just above interventricular septum and medial to the opening of the coronary sinus.

The heart is a **four-chambered muscular pump**. The *right side* pumps blood to the lungs for oxygenation (lesser circuit), and the *left side* pumps the oxygenated blood to the organs and tissues of the body (systemic or greater circuit). The heart also has **endocrine** functions by producing the hormone *atrial natriuretic peptide* (ANP) for the regulation of water and salt homeostasis. The **systole** is the contraction, and the **diastole** the dilatation (relaxation) of the heart muscle. We distinguish an *atrial* and *a ventricular systole*, and an *atrial* and *a ventricular diastole*. The ventricular systole has two phases: In the 1st phase, all cuspid and semilunar valves are closed, and the ventricle is able to increase the pressure in its chamber called an isovolumetric contraction (blood volume remains constant, pressure increases). In the 2nd phase, the pressure in the ventricles passes the pressure in the aorta and pulmonary trunk, and pushes the aortic and pulmonary valves open. The **1st heart sound** corresponds to the beginning of the ventricular systole, and is the consequence of the contraction of the heart muscle. The **2nd heart sound** results from the closure of the aortic and pulmonary valves, which can be heard best at the right and left 2nd intercostal spaces, respectively.

Heart muscle cells (*cardiomyocytes*, striated muscle) are electrically coupled through gap junctions (intercalated discs) & show spontanous electrical activity that is under the control of the electrical conducting system of the heart (sinoatrial & atrioventricular nodes, His-bundles, Purkinje-fibres). Thus, the heart muscle is a functional syncytium. Its action is modulated by the autonomic nervous system.

- **Lungs, pleura and pleural cavities**

- View the **parietal pleura** covering the lt. and rt. pleural cavities with its *costal, diaphragmatic* and *mediastinal parts*. Study the extensions of the pleural space named costodiaphragmatic and *costomediastinal* recesses, and *oesophageal recess* (on the right only). The so-called *pulmonary ligaments* are formed at the **junction** *of the visceral and parietal pleurae*.

- Inspect the **visceral pleura** attached to the surface of the lungs. View the **lobules** separated by the *interlobular septa*, which can be seen particularly well in smokers and/or persons, who lived in an air-poluted environment, because the "dirty particles" from the air are phagocytosed and stored in the septa (lymphatic drainage).

- Now study the *apex, hilum, fissures* and *lobes* of the **rt. and lt. lungs**. Inspect the **topographical relationship** of the lungs to neighbouring structures by looking at the impression of thoracic structures on the surface of lungs (azygous vein, sup. vena cava, brachiocephalic veins, aorta, subclavian artery, oesophagus, cardiac impression and cardiac notch).

- In the **hilum** of the lungs follow/dissect the *course of arteries together with bronchi*, and inspect the *separate course of veins in the interlobular septa*.

- View the different positions of the *pulmonary arteries, main bronchi* and *pulmonary veins* at the **rt. and lt. pulmonary hilum,** and identify them by their consistency (*on the right*: right sup. lobar branch upon the pulmonary artery, *on the left*: pulmonary artery above the main left bronchus).

The **lungs** are spongy organs essential for **gas exchange** consisting of *bronchi, bronchioli, alveoli, blood and lymph vessels, visceral nerves (vagal afferents* for stretch receptors, *autonomic afferents* for blood circulation and bronchial constriction/dilation*)* and *connective tissue*. All **bronchi** and **bronchioli** branch dichotomely into two branches at one branching point. The rt. and lt. *main bronchi* give rise to **lobar bronchi**, and these to **segment bronchi**. Segment bronchi branch off several times before they become *bronchioli*. Bronchioli further branch dichotomely, until they form *terminal bronchioli* supplying a **lobule** of the lung. Eventually, they discharge into *alveolar ducts* and *alveoli* (small air-filled chambers). Bronchi differ from bronchioli in their epithelium, and thickness of their walls made up by smooth muscle and cartilage (see **Histology**). The alveoli and respiratory bronchioli (alveolar ducts) are sites of gas exchange.

Bronchi and bronchioli **course together** *with arteries*, whereas the *veins course together with lymph vessels* in the connective tissue separating divisions of the lung (*interlobular, intersegmental*, and *interlobar septa*). At the hilum of the lung, a second lymphatic drainage pathway starting blind at and coursing together with bronchi joins the lymphatic drainage originating in the septa.

The **right main** bronchus is in **continuation with the trachea** almost in a straight line. This is why it is more likely that an object like a nut or *extracted tooth* falls into your right main bronchus rather than into your left main bronchus.

- **Diaphragm and respiration**

- Identify the **central tendon** (*site of insertion*), and the **costal, sternal and lumbar origins** of the diaphragm. View the *sternocostal triangle*, the *rt. and lt. crus of the lumbar part* of the diaphragm, and the *rt. and lt. domes* (right dome is higher).

- Many structures of the mediastinum pass through the diaphragm **on their way** from the thorax to the abdomen. Trace following **structures passing through the diaphragm**: *Aorta and thoracic duct, oesophagus with ant. and post. vagal plexus*, the *sympathetic chain* (or *sympathetic trunk*), the *greater, lesser, and least splanchnic nerves*, and the *ascending lumbar veins* (their continuation in the thorax are the azygous and hemiazygous veins).

The diaphragm is the most important **muscle of respiration** consisting of costal, sternal and lumbar parts, which all insert at the central tendon of the diaphragm. Upon contraction, the muscular parts of the diaphragm pull the central tendon inferiorly, and facilitate **inspiration**. On the thoracic site, the pericardial sac of the heart it attached to the central tendon.

During inspiration, the volume of the **thoracic cage** increases through the *contraction of muscles of inspiration*, which causes a *negative pressure* in the *pleural cavities*. Because the lungs are elastic organs filled with air (*compressible*), whereas the pleural cavities are filled with a very thin layer of serous liquid (*non-compressible*), the lungs follow the movement of the thoracic cage during inspiration, and suck in air. The **principal muscles of inspiration** are the *diaphragm* (abdominal or belly breathing), and the *external intercostal* muscles working together with the *interchondral part* (=intercartilaginous) of the *internal intercostal* muscles (enlargement of thoracic cage in transverse axis). **Accessory muscles of inspiration** are mainly the *sternocleidomastoid* and *ant., middle and post. scalene* muscles, but the *trapezius* and *levator scapulae* muscles can also contribute to inspiration (all muscles lift the thoracic cage, enlargement in sagittal axis).

In contrast, **quiet expiration** is a **passive** process, in which the muscles of inspiration relax and the volume of the thoracic cage returns back to its original size. This results in an increase of pressure in the pleural cavities, and recoil of lung tissue. **Muscles of active expiration** are the *internal intercostal* muscles (*except* the interchondral part), and *abdominal muscles* (rectus abdominis, external oblique, internal oblique and transversus abdominis muscles, see **Body Wall**), which can all move the thoracic cage downward. The *latissimus dorsi* muscle is a **muscle of forced expiration** (if arms are fixed, often used by asthmatic patients who suffer from bronchoconstriction and emphysema).

Pneumothorax is a pathological condition, in which air fills in the pleural cavity. The air can enter the pleural cavity from *outside* through damage to the thoracic wall (e.g. traumatic injury) or from *inside* through damage to bronchi or lung tissue (e.g. rupture of cystic alveolar dilatations of lung tissue in *bullous emphysema* or spontaneous pneumothorax mainly in young males).

16. ABDOMEN AND PELVIS

In the **abdomen**, we will **view** the subregions of the *abdominal cavity*, and abdominal *organs* with their *attachments, topographical relationship* to neighbouring structures, and their *blood and nerve supply*. We will also note the **pelvic** *organs* and the *pelvic and urogenital diaphragms*.

16.1 PROSECTIONS AND MODELS

Hepar = Liver, Gaster = stomach, Lien = spleen, Ren = kidney

- **Abdominal surface markings and regions**
- Identify the borders of the rt. and lt. *hypochondrium, epigastrium*, rt. and lt. *flanks*, rt. and lt. *umbilical regions, hypogastrium*.

- **Overview of the peritoneal cavity**
- In the **abdominal cavity** first view the **parietal** and **visceral peritoneum**.
- View the **lesser and greater omentum** formed by the *hepatogastric and hepatoduodenal ligaments*, the structures coursing in the hepatoduodenal ligament reaching the *hilum of the liver* (*proper hepatic artery, portal vein, bile duct*), and the *epiploic (omental) foramen* dorsal to the hepatoduodenal ligament, which is the entrance of the omental bursa (see below).
- Identify the abdominal part of the **oesophagus** and the *cardia* (transition to the stomach) with the cardiac notch of the **stomach**. View the *lesser and greater curvatures, fundus, body, pyloric antrum* and *pyloric canal* of the stomach. Palpate the *pyloric sphincter*.
- Identify the **liver, spleen,** and **small and large intestines** with their **mesenteries** as well as the **rectum and anal canal**.
- The **small intestine** contains the *duodenum, jejunum* and *ileum*. The duodenum is secondarily retroperitoneal except for its superior part, whereas the jejunum and ileum are intraperitoneal beginning from the *duodenojejunal flexure*.
- The **large intestine** (*colon*) can be identified by the taeniae coli (longitudinal muscles), appendices epiploicae and haustrae (which reflect the contraction status of the colon at death like a snap-shot). The colon consists of the *cecum* with the *appendix vermiformis, ascending colon, transverse colon, descending colon, sigmoid colon* and *rectum*. Among these divisions, the ascending and descending colon became attached to the dorsal body wall together with their mesenteries in development, and *secondarily retroperitoneal* (or partially intraperitoneal, because they can be accessed from the peritoneal cavity).
- Open the **omental bursa** & view the structures localised at its anterior/posterior, cranial/caudal, right/left **walls** (important to *understand pancreatic disease*):

Anteriorly, you will find the liver and stomach with the lesser omentum in-between, and the gastro-colic part of the greater omentum connecting the stomach with the transverse colon.

Posteriorly, inspect the pancreas, aorta with coeliac trunk, inf. vena cava, lumbar part of diaphragm as well as the left suprarenal gland and pole of kidney. The cisterna chyli (= sac at origin of thoracic duct) is hidden between the aorta and inf. vena cava.

On the *right* border you will again see the liver, and on the *left* the spleen as well as the gastro-splenic, phrenico-colic, and spleno-renal ligaments.

The omental bursa extends *cranially* towards the diaphragm and gastro-phrenic ligaments, and *caudally* to the transverse mesocolon. The *pockets* of the omental bursa are the superior recess (between aorta and vena cava), inferior recess (between ant. and post. layers of greater omentum) and lateral (splenic) recess.

- The **pancreas** localised at the dorsal wall of the omental bursa can be *accessed* from intraabdominally by transecting the transverse mesocolon, gastro-colic ligament or hepato-gastric part of the lesser omentum.

- **Other recesses and spaces** in the abdominal cavity are the

  duodenal recesses (at the duodenojejunal flexure)

  caecal recesses (at the caecum),

  intersigmoid recess,

  rt. & lt. subphrenic spaces,

  rt. & lt. paracolic gutters (between body wall and ascending and descending colon, respectively)

  and *rt. & lt. mesocolic spaces* (between the mesentery of the small intestine and colon).

The inflammation of the peritoneum is called **peritonitis**, which is a serious life-threatening condition, if not treated immediately. An intraperitoneal infection can also be restricted to pouches, recesses, gutters, and other spaces of the abdominal cavity, e.g. a subphrenic abscess (pus in the subphrenic space).

- There are **three major trunks or arteries of the gut** in line with the development of its divisions:

  (1) The **celiac trunk** supplies all structures deriving from the foregut (liver, stomach, duodenum, pancreas) or developing in its mesenteries (spleen).

  (2) The **superior mesenteric artery** supplies structures deriving from the midgut (duodenum, pancreas, jejunum, ileum, cecum and appendix, ascending colon, proximal 2/3rds of transverse colon).

  (3) The **inferior mesenteric artery** supplies structures deriving from the hindgut (distal 1/3rd of transverse colon, descending colon, sigmoid colon, upper portion of rectum).

The duodenum and pancreas positioned at the junction of the foregut and midgut are supplied by both the *celiac trunk* and *superior mesenteric artery.*

The proximal two-thirds of the transverse colon (located on the right side *except in situs inversus*) are still part of the midgut, whereas the distal (left) one-third of the transverse colon belongs to the hindgut. Please note that in addition to the changes in blood supply at the midgut- hindgut- junction (**Connon-Boehm**), the hindgut is **not supplied** by the *vagus nerve* anymore like the derivatives of the whole foregut and midgut, but it receives its parasympathetic innervation from the *sacral spinal cord.*

- **Overview of retroperitoneal organs and structures**
- View the following **primarily retroperitoneal** structures in the **retroperitoneal space**:

  the *abdominal aorta* and *inf. vena cava*

  common iliac vessels <u>and</u> their division into the *external & internal iliac vessels*

  rt. & lt. *suprarenal glands* and *kidneys* with their blood supply

  psoas major and *quadratus lumborum muscles*

  lumbar plexus (iliohypogastric nerve, ilioinguinal nerve, genitofemoral nerve, lateral cutaneous nerve of thigh, femoral nerve, obturator nerve)

  rt. & lt. *segmental vessels* of the body wall (<u>paired</u>)

  sympathetic chain with paired paravertebral ganglia and ganglion impar (= unpaired ganglion)

  lymph nodes (so far preserved)

- **Portal-systemic anastomoses**
- Now we will study the **portal-systemic (portal-caval) anastomoses**, which connect the portal vein with the sup. & inf. vena cava through veins in the ventral body wall, pelvis, thorax and retroperitoneum.

  paraumbilical veins in the round ligament of the liver (connected to the veins in the subcutaneous fatty layer around the umbilicus)

  superior rectal vein (connected to the middle and inf. rectal veins)

  lt. gastric vein (connected to esophageal veins)

  and veins of secondarily retroperitoneal organs (connected to segmental veins of the posterior body wall)

The portal-systemic anatomoses (portacaval anastomoses) become important, when the **portal vein is obstructed**. Due to the high pressure in the portal venous system, the blood surpasses the liver and other organs drained by the portal vein, and flows directly into the branches of the inf. and sup. vena cava.

The high pressure in the collateral circuits draining the blood through the porto-caval anastomosis can cause a **venous bleeding** especially from *oesophageal veins*, which is often life-threatening, or from *rectal veins* (haemorrhoids).

The *direct flow* of the blood from the middle and inf. rectal veins into the *inf. vena cava* becomes important, when patients receive a **suppository** (e.g. pain killer after tooth extraction). Drugs applied in this way usually act very quickly, because they **by-passes the liver** without being metabolised there.

- **Major organs**

Liver and gallbladder

In order to understand the functional anatomy of the liver, we will have to study first the gross anatomy of the liver.

- View the **four lobes of the liver** called the *right, left, quadrate* and *caudate lobes*. The lobes are further divided into **segments**, which are particularly important for liver surgery, e.g. cysts or cancer restricted to liver segments can be cured by removing these segments.
- In the **hilum**, inspect the *proper hepatic artery*, *portal vein* and the *lt. and rt. hepatic ducts* forming the *common hepatic duct*. Find also the common hepatic duct, which joins the *cystic duct* of the gallbladder to form the *common bile duct*.
- Trace the course of the **common bile** duct from the *hepatoduodenal ligament* to the *retroduodenal space, pancreatic tissue* and wall of the duodenum. View the *common channel* with the *main pancreatic duct* (if present) and the opening into the duodenum at the *major duodenal papilla (Vater)*.
- Find the **bare area of liver** not covered by peritoneum, and the *coronary* and *triangular ligaments*. View the attachment of the **gallbladder** to the liver, and the visceral peritoneum covering the abdominal surface of the gallbladder.
- Find the *falciform ligament* and *round ligament* (ligamentum teres hepatis), which are parts of the ventral mesentery like the lesser omentum.

The liver is a *derivative of the duodenum* (budding of foregut). It is a highly active **metabolic organ**, which also **synthesizes** important *blood proteins* (albumin, blood clotting proteins, etc.). Thus, *liver failure* causes, among other deficits like ammonia intoxication, also oedema due to hypoosmolarity in blood (low colloid osmotic pressure resulting from hypoalbuminemia), and an increased bleeding tendency. Portal hypertension in liver cirrhosis causes **ascites** (fluid in peritoneal cavity). Because the **portal vein** carries all nutrients taken up by the gut first to the liver (except for fatty acids transported by the thoracic duct), the liver is the **first station** in the metabolisation of food and inactivation of drugs. Thus, only substances, which pass the liver at the first instance, reach the general circulation.

The liver is also a **gland**, which secrets **bile**. Degradation products, poisons and *conjugated* molecules (e.g. drugs or bilirubin) are excreted into the same bile duct system. The bile is stored and concentrated in the gallbladder. The bile acids are **recycled**, because after their secretion they are re-absorbed by the gut and brought back to the liver via the portal vein, where they are secreted again, etc. This whole process is called the *entoro-hepatic cycle*. In contrast, molecules, which are not recycled, e.g. inactivated drugs, are excreted.

In 70% of cases, the bile duct and main pancreatic duct drain together into the duodenum at the *major duodenal papilla*. If then the common channel of the bile and pancreatic ducts is obstructed (e.g. by a gall stone), the skin of the patients becomes yellowish, which is called **jaundice**.

Spleen
- View the topographical relationship of the spleen to related organs. Inspect the **margins** and **hilum** of the spleen including its **vessels**.
- View a **cross section** of the spleen. Try to differentiate the *red and white pulp*, which can be seen easier in an unfixed (fresh) spleen (see also **Histology**).

The spleen is a *lymphoreticular organ*, and the only lymphatic organ **filtering bacteria directly from blood**. In patients, who have no spleen (after splenectomy), the risk of a *sepsis* (blood poisoning by bacteria) is higher, especially for certain types of microbes (e.g. pneumococcal bacteria). Please note that such bacteria can invade the blood system easily from anywhere in the body, and also from *infected teeth*. The lymphatic tissue is localised in the **white pulp** of the spleen.

The **red pulp** of the spleen filters and **eliminates old erythrocytes** from blood. The *splenic vein*, which drains into the portal vein, brings *degradation products* of erythrocytes *back to liver* for their excretion together with bile (e.g. bilirubin).

With its sponge-like structure, the spleen can also **store blood**, and return it to the blood circulation by active contraction.

Pancreas
- Study the **head**, **body** and **tail** of the pancreas in the retroperitoneal space at the bottom of the omental bursa.
- Inspect the head of the pancreas located in the C of the duodenum and separated by the superior mesenteric vessels into the uncinate process and a dorsal portion.
- View the course of the **main and accessory ducts** of the pancreas during their course in pancreatic tissue and their openings into the duodenum.

At the *foregut/midgut junction* (becomes the duodenum), the pancreas develops out of two buds, which fuse to form the pancreas. The *dorsal bud* generates most of the pancreas, whereas the *ventral bud* arises beside the bile duct and forms only some parts of the pancreatic head and the uncinate process. Therefore, the main and accessory ducts, originating from the ventral and dorsal buds respectively, may join or drain separately into the duodenum. The pancreas has an **exocrine** part, which excretes its *enzymes into the duodenum* through the main and accessory ducts for *digestion of molecules* (carbohydrates, lipids, proteins, nucleic acids), and an **endocrine** part, which produces *hormones* and secretes them *into the blood* (insulin, glucagon, somatostatin). You can see the endocrine part of the pancreas only under the microscope (islets of Langerhans).

71

Kidneys, ureters, urinary bladder and suprarenal glands

- View the **two kidneys and suprarenal glands** in the retroperitoneal space. The left kidney lies more cranially than the right kidney.

- Inspect the *renal fascia*, the *perirenal fat* and the *fibrous capsule* attached to the **surface of the kidney**. Identify the **hilum** and there the *renal artery, renal vein* and *ureter*. The **renal sinus** contains fat in continuity with the *perirenal fat* and the branches of renal blood vessels.

- In a **kidney sectioned**, you will be able to view the *renal cortex, renal medulla,* and *renal calices* in continuity with the *renal pelvis* and *ureter*. The cortex of the kidney reaches the base of the pyramids at the border to the renal medulla, and these extensions of the renal cortex called renal column are located between individual pyramids. The *pyramids* of the *renal medulla* emerge as *renal papilla* into the *minor calices* to pour the urine into calices.

- View the **urinary bladder** fixed at the ant. portion of the pelvic arch (inner aspect of pubic bones) and the entry of the ureter into the bladder. The urinary bladder only expands cranially and posteriorly, when it is filled with urine.

- View the **lt. and rt. renal arteries** and **veins**. Inspect the **three suprarenal arteries** (from the inferior phrenic artery, directly from the aorta, and from the renal artery, respectively).

The **kidney** is an important organ required for **filtering blood** and excretion of degradation products into the urine. It consists of 5 **segments** and 7-14 **lobules**, the latter of which are separate lobules (renculi) in the human fetus, before they fuse. In the adult kidney, the junctions between the lobules become the renal columns, because each lobule has a cortex around a pyramid-shaped medulla.

A **nephron** is the basic anatomical and functional unit of the kidney consisting of a *glomerulus, proximal convoluted tubule, loop of Henle* and *distal convoluted tubule*. The most distal portion of the nephrons – the distal convoluted tubule - is connected through a *connecting tubule* to a *collecting tubule*, which eventually discharges the urine into the *minor calyx*. The urine further flows into the *major calyx, renal pelvis* and *ureter*, and from there into *urinary bladder*, where it is stored. During micturition, the stored urine leaves the urinary bladder, and is discharged through the *urethra* (see pelvic cavity below).

The distal convoluted tubule approaches the *vascular pole of the glomerulus* of the same nephron, before it connects to a connecting tubule. The contact point is the **juxtaglomerular apparatus**, which is critical for regulating the renal blood flow and glomerular filtration rate of primary urine. Please note that the *loop of Henle* is that part of the nephron, which consists of the proximal straight tubule extending from the renal cortex to the medulla, the intermediary tubule in the medulla and the distal tubule coursing back from the medulla to the cortex (see also **Histology** and **Physiology** books).

Kidneys also **produce hormones** (e.g. *erythropoietin* and *prostaglandins*) or activate them. For example, the kidneys activate the prehormone 25-hydroxy-Vitamin D (*calcidiol*) by metabolising it into 1,25-dihydroxy-Vitamine D (*calcitriol*) to enhance to calcium uptake in the gut. In addition, *renin* produced in the juxtaglomerular apparatus of the kidney is an enzyme that cleaves the prehormone angiotensinogen I, and is a part of the *renin-angiotensin-system* important for the regulation of the blood pressure.

The **suprarenal glands** are organs neighbouring the kidneys (located on their upper pole). They have a *cortex* producing *steroid hormones*, and a *medulla* functioning as a sympathetic ganglion, which produces *adrenalin* and *noradrenalin* (see also **Histology**).

- **Overview of pelvic cavity**

- The **pelvic floor** is formed by the levator ani muscle (*pelvic diaphragm*) and the perineal muscles (part of *urogenital diaphragm*).

- In the **pelvic cavity**, view the following structures:

  branches of the *internal* and *external iliac arteries* and *veins* (e.g. supplying urinary bladder, uterus, ovaries, prostate, rectum, gluteal region, etc.)

  the sacral plexus,

  contents of the pelvic cavity in *females* including the urinary bladder, uterus, uterine tubes, ovaries, rectum, utero-vesical and recto-uterine pouches (pouch of Douglas).

  contents of the pelvic cavity in *males* including the urinary bladder, rectum and vesiculo-rectal pouch.

Ovaries are not only the site of production of the female eggs cells (ovum) undergoing different cycles. They also produce different amounts of *steroid hormones* (*oestrogene, progesterone*) depending on the stage of the oestrous cycle.

In males, the **testes** produce sperms and *steroid hormones* (e.g. *testosterone*).

The **urethra of men** is a common duct for sperms (with secrections of the seminal vesicles, prostate gland and bulbourethral glands) as well as urine coursing from the bladder through the penis. The prostate of men is localised below the urinary bladder around the urethra, and can obstruct the urethra in prostate cancer.

The **urethra of females** is shorter than in males. Therefore, ascending urinary infections affecting the urinary bladder are more common in females than in males.

17. UPPER LIMB

In the **upper limb**, we will pay special attention to the shoulder and axillary region, and to the arm, because of the **close proximity of these regions to the neck**. They contain many structures coming from or coursing to the neck including blood and lymph vessels, and nerves. The **superficial veins**, the **radial artery** and the **deltoid muscle** are particularly important for *intravenous injections, measuring the arterial pulse* and *intramuscular injections,* respectively.

17.1 PROSECTIONS AND MODELS

- **Bones**

- Identify the *acromial* and *sternal ends* of the **clavicle**.

- Inspect the *costal* and *dorsal surfaces*, and the *lateral, medial* and *superior borders* of the **scapula**, as well as its *angles, spine, glenoid fossa, coracoid process, acromion,* and *main muscular attachments*.

- The head of the **humerus** forms the *shoulder joint* together with the *glenoid fossa of the scapula*. View the *greater* and *lesser tuberosities* of the humerus and the *deltoid tuberosity*, which are insertion points for shoulder muscles. The *bicipital groove* contains the tendon of the long head of the biceps brachii muscle, and the *radial groove* the radial nerve. The *med. and lat. epicondyles* are the common origin of several flexor and extensor muscles. View also the relationship of the *olecranon* to the ulnar nerve.

- View the bones of the forearm. In supination (anatomical position), the **radius** is the *lateral bone* (proximal and distal ends, head, neck, tuberosity), and the **ulna** is the *medial bone* (proximal and distal ends, head, coronoid process, olecranon, styloid processes).

- Note that **carpal bones** form one **proximal row** (scaphoid, lunate, triquetral, pisiform) and one **distal row** (trapezium, trapezoid, capitate, hamate).

- In the hand, we have **metacarpals** and **phalanges** giving rise to the fingers (2 phalanges in the thumb, and 3 phalanges in all other fingers).

- View the *shoulder, elbow* and *wrist* **joints** including their articular surfaces and main ligaments. They are all synovial joints. Identify the hinge joints and the ball and socket varieties as examples for different joint forms.

The **axillary nerve** coursing around the neck of the humerus can be damaged by *humeral dislocations* and by *fractures at the surgical neck*. The **radial nerve** is normally protected in the *radial groove* at the shaft of the humerus, but it can be damaged by *fractures of the humerus shaft* because of the close proximity to the bone.

- **Shoulder girdle**

- Inspect the **muscles acting at the shoulder girdle** including the pectoralis major and minor, subclavius, serratus ant., latissimus dorsi, trapezius, rhomboid major and minor, and levator scapulae muscles. These muscles are innervated directly by the *brachial plexus (mostly supraclavicular branches)* except for the trapezius muscle, which is innervated by both the 11th cranial nerve (accessory nerve) and posterior rami of superior cervical spinal nerves (C2-C4).

- Identify the four **rotator cuff muscles** stabilising the *capsule of the shoulder joint*: the *supraspinatus and infraspinatus muscles* (innervated by the suprascapular nerve), the *teres minor muscle* (innervated by the axillary nerve) and the *subscapularis muscle* (innervated by the subscapular nerve). The *teres major muscle* (innervated by the thoracodorsal or lower subscapular nerve) does not belong the rotator cuff muscles, because it does not support or strengthen the capsule of the shoulder joint.

- **Brachial plexus and axilla**

- The **brachial plexus** is a nerve plexus supplying the upper limb. It is formed by the ventral rami of the lower cervical (C5-C8) and the first thoracic (T1) spinal nerves.

  (a) Study the ***main portion*** of the brachial plexus with its:

  roots (continuation of ventral rami of spinal nerves C5-T1, because developmentally the upper limb is the extension of the ventral body wall; *CAVE:* unlucky terminology, do not mix up with the "ventral and dorsal roots of the spinal nerves" connected to the spinal cord),

  trunks (superior trunk from C5-6*, middle trunk* from C7*, inferior trunk* from C8-T1*),*

  divisions that form the cords (ant. divisions the medial & lateral cords, post. divisions the posterior cord),

  cords (*lateral cord* from sup. & middle trunks, *medial cord* from inferior trunk, *posterior cord* from all tree trunks - through divisions mentioned above),

  (b) Note that the ***supraclavicular branches*** of the brachial plexus can originate from the roots, trunks or cords: *suprascapular, subscapular, thoracodorsal* (=dorsal scapular), *subclavian, pectoralis major & minor,* and *long thoracic* nerves.

  (c) Study the ***infraclavicular branches*** (*terminal branches*) of the brachial plexus formed by the cords supplying arm, forearm and wrist/hand (see below).

- The **axilla** is a *pyramid-shaped* space with its base at the skin and superficial fascia of the armpit <u>connected to the neck</u>. The borders of the axilla formed:

  (a) **anteriorly** by the *clavicle, pectoralis major* and *pectoralis minor* muscles, **laterally** by the *humerus* and *arm flexors,* **medially** by the *serratus anterior muscle* and the *thoracic wall,* and **posteriorly** by the *latissimus dorsi muscle, scapula* and *subscapularis muscle.*

(b) Learn the **contents** of the axilla including the *brachial plexus, axillary artery & vein*, and the *axillary lymph vessels* and *lymph nodes*. You may not be able to see many lymph nodes, but try to localise the **superficial and deep stations** of lymph nodes and discuss the **convergence of lymphatic drainage** from the superficial chest (including the breast) with lymph vessels of the arm.

- **Arm**
- In the arm, identify the **deltoid muscle** innervated by the *axillary nerve*, the **flexor muscles** innervated by the *musculocutaneous nerve* (biceps, coracobrachialis, brachialis), and the **extensor muscle** innervated by the *radial nerve* (triceps).
- The **medial triangular space** is surrounded by the teres minor (proximally) and major (distally) muscles and long arm of the triceps muscle (laterally) transmitting the *circumflex scapular artery*.
- The borders of the **lateral quadrangular space** are the humerus (laterally), the long arm of the triceps (medially), the teres minor (proximally) and teres major (distally) transmitting the axillary nerve and posterior circumflex humeral artery.

> **Intramuscular injections** into the **deltoid muscle** should be avoided at the back of the arm, because then structures in the lateral quadrangular space can be lesioned.

- **Cubital fossa**
- First identify the *cephalic, basilic,* and *median cubital* **veins**, and follow their course.
- Next identify the **boundaries of the cubital fossa** and view the arrangement of nerves, veins and arteries by considering that you give an *intravenous injection*.

- **Forearm**
- View the **superficial flexors**, which have a common origin at the medial epicondyle (*palmaris longus, flexor carpi radialis & ulnaris, humeral head of pronator teres*), the **intermediate flexor** (*flexor digitorum superficialis*), and the **deep flexors** of the forearm (*flexor policis longus, pronator quadratus, flexor digitorum profundus*).
- View the **innervation** of the forearm flexors by the *median nerve*. Note that the two ulnar divisions of the flexor digitorum profundus for the flexion of the 4th- 5th fingers and the flexor carpi ulnaris are not innervated by the median nerve but the ulnar nerve.
- View the **superficial extensor muscles** (*brachioradialis, extensor carpi radialis longus & brevis, extensor digitorum, extensor digiti minimi*), and the **deep extensor muscles** of the forearm (*supinator, abductor policis longus, extensor policis longus & brevis, extensor indices*); all extensor muscles are **innervated** by the *radial nerve*.

Fascias of the forearm form **tight compartments**, which do not allow an extension if there is *muscle damage* or *bleeding* within the fascia called *compartment syndrome*. In the long term, this can result in a total atrophy and palsy of muscles in the compartment involved. Please note that **complex regional pain syndromes** (*CRPS, neuropathic pain, Sudeck*) can lead to similar symptoms including *numbness*, *painful sensations*, and *motor palsies* of the forearm and hand, as well as *autonomic disturbances* (changes in sweating, blood flow, temperature regulation, oedema, etc.). Although the pathophysiology of the latter syndromes is not totally understood, they can be treated with a **blockade of the sympathetic nervous system at the stellate ganglion (see Pharynx Practical** for more information).

- **Wrist and hand**

- View the **flexor retinaculum** and structures coursing *upon and below the retinaculum*. A *carpal tunnel syndrome* is damage to the *median nerve* under the flexor retinaculum. Therefore, the sensory and motor innervation are affected only more distally including the opponens and abductor pollicis breves muscles and the sensory regions of the hand innervated by the median nerve.

- View the **palmar aponeurosis**. The palmaris longus muscle located superficially to the aponeurosis is not always present.

- View the **thenar and hpothenar,** and **interossei and lumbrical muscles** innervated by the median and ulnar nerves.

- Inspect the **cutaneous nerve supply** of the hand following the *branches of the radial nerve (dorsally)* as well as the *median and ulnar nerves (ventrally, palmar)*. Hereby consider that you may need to puncture a vein at the dorsum of the hand.

A **Dupuytren's contracture** is a shortening and thickening of the longitudinal bands of the palmar aponeurosis caused by fibrosis. In addition, the longitudinal bands of the palmar aponeurosis may become fixed to the tendons of long forearm flexor muscles. The fibrous degeneration of the longitudinal bands of the palmar aponeurosis can pull the fingers into partial flexion (usually the ring and little fingers affected).

A **'claw hand'** is the result of an *ulnar nerve lesion* that leads to a paralysis of the ulnar lumbrical (flex in metacarpophalangeal joints, stretch the fingers) and interossei muscles (adduct & abduct fingers towards middle finger, assist lumbricals). A **'wrist drop'** occurs, when the *main branch of the radial nerve* is damaged (often combined with a pronation & flexion of the forearm). An **'ape hand'** results from a *median nerve damage* at the level the pronator teres muscle, which becomes evident, when the patient tries to make a fist, because the two divisions of the flexor digitorum profundus innervated by the ulnar nerve can still flex the 4th and 5th fingers. However, the 2nd and 3rd fingers innervated by the median nerve cannot be flexed.

You should know that a lesion of the *brachial plexus* at the *neck or axilla* can lead to similar palsies, e.g. upper and lower plexus lesions (Erb-Duchenne palsy, Dejerine-Klumpke palsy). Such plexus lesions usually occur after a **trauma** but can also result from **infections** *descending from the head to the neck* or space occupying **tumours** in the neck.

Moreover, **general infections of the nervous system** can result in a paralysis of many topographically related or unrelated peripheral nerves and subregions of a plexus (e.g. following a polyradiculitis caused by a borrelliosis). Likewise widespread sensory and motor symptoms can be encountered in **neuropathies**, e.g. in diabetic neuropathy (including nerves in upper limb, head & neck).

- **Blood supply and taking the pulse**

- Look at the positions of the *axillary*, *brachial*, *ulnar* and *radial arteries* considering that you have to **take the pulse** of a patient, and note that there are several collateral circulations in the arm. A normal *radial pulse* rate should be in a range between 60-80 beats per minute.

- The **radial artery** is often used to directly **collect arterial blood** (to determine the level of blood gases and analyse the function of the lungs), or the **place an arterial catheter** (*arterial blood samples*, *blood pressure monitoring* during anaesthesia or in intensive care units). However, it is recommended to perform an *Allen's test* (or Doppler ultrasound) before puncturing the radial artery to test for the patency of collateral circulation between the radial and ulnar arteries. [The patient makes a tight fist, while the examiner compresses the radial or ulnar artery. If the hand turns pink after the patient opens the hand (while examiner still keeps pressing the artery), the anastomosis between both vessels is sufficient.]

- View the **deep veins** (*axillary*, *brachial*, *radial* and *ulnar veins*), and recapitulate the course of the **main superficial veins** discharging into the brachial vein (*cephalic vein*), and axillary vein (*basilic vein*). Study the *medial cubital vein*, the *medial antebrachial veins*, and the *dorsal venous arch on the back of the hand* used for venipuncture.

If you perform a **paravenous injection** (injection missing or severely puncturing the vein, pumping of syringe content into the connective tissue around the vein) and/or the injection site becomes **infected**, the neighbouring nerves may be damaged (higher likelihood of infection in paravenous injection).
In the cubital fossa, the nerves that can be affected are the *posterior cutaneous nerve of forearm* (from radial nerve), *lateral cutaneous nerve of forearm* (from musculocutaneous nerve) and *medial cutaneous nerve of forearm* (directly from the medial cord of the brachial plexus), whereas in the hand you may damage *branches of the radial nerve*. **Therefore, study the borders of regions receiving their sensory innervation from these nerves thoroughly!**

18. NEUROANATOMY - I

We will first view the divisions of the **brain and spinal cord**. In a next step, we will then study the **brainstem** with the **cranial nerves**, the **cerebellum**, and the **meninges** and **blood supply** of the nervous system.

18.1 DISSECTIONS

- **Dissection of blood vessels of the brain**
- First identify the **arachnoid mater**. It is a milky membrane on the brain surface, which does not follow the contours of the gyri and sulci. In the fixed brains, it is collapsed, because the cerebrospinal fluid (CSF) diffuses out of the subarachnoid space that is localised below the arachnoid membrane.
- Remove the arachnoid membrane gently from **dorsal portions** of the cerebral hemispheres, brainstem and cerebellum.
- **Ventrally (basis of brain)**, find the major blood vessels supplying the brain. These are the **vertebral & basilar arteries** (posterior circuit), and the **internal carotid artery with its branches** (anterior circuit). The ant. and post. circuits are connected through the arterial **circle of Willis**.
- Dissect the blood vessels with their major branches carefully from the brain surface, and free them from the arachnoid membrane.
- Take a **polystyrene plate**, and pin the various branches of the anterior and posterior circuits together with the **circle of Willis** on the plate. **Study them carefully** (see branches below **in Prosections & Models**).

18.2 PROSECTIONS AND MODELS

- **Divisions of the adult nervous system**
- The two main divisions of the **central nervous system** (**CNS**) are the **brain** and the **spinal cord.**

   (a) In the brain, identify the *telencephalon, diencephalon, mesencephalon* (midbrain), *metencephalon* (pons + cerebellum) & *myeloencephalon* (medulla).

   (b) In the spinal cord, find the *cervical* (C1-8), *thoracic* (T1-T12), *lumbar* (L1-L5), and *sacral* (S1-5) segments, and the *coccygeal* segment. They can be identified with the aid of the ventral (ant.) and dorsal (post.) roots forming the spinal nerves of the respective segments. Inspect also the course of the spinal nerves in the *intervertebral foramina*.

- The **peripheral nervous system** (**PNS**) consists of **nerves** (*spinal, cranial* and *visceral nerves*) and **ganglia**, the latter term referring to a group of neurons in the periphery (*spinal ganglia, cranial nerve ganglia*, and *autonomic ganglia*). The PNS has both somatic (somatic nervous system, SNS) and autonomic components (autonomic nervous system, ANS).

- **Divisions of the developing nervous system**
- View the **neural tube** (four week old human embryo), and the **developing brain** (eight week old human fetus) with the *rhombencephalon* (for myelo- & metencephalon), *mesencephalon* and *prosencephalon* (for di- & telencephalon).

- **Spinal cord and spinal nerve**
- View the *cervical and lumbar enlargements* of the spinal cord for the *brachial and lumbar plexus*, respectively. Note that in *adults* the spinal cord only reaches to the segment L2, and ends with the *conus medullaris* here. View the *cauda equina*, (made of ventral and dorsal roots for spinal nerves) and the *filum terminale* (continuation of the spinal cord out of connective tissue).
- Study horizontal sections through the spinal cord at different segments. First, orientate yourself by identifying the *ventral median fissure* (lies anteriorly) and the *dorsal median sulcus* (lies posteriorly). Now identify the *gray matter* (groupings of neurons) forming the so-called "horns", and the *white matter tracts* that surround the horns. Inspect the butterfly shape of the spinal cord with the *rt. & lt. ventral horns*, and the *rt. & lt. dorsal horns*. At the segments T1 to L2 / 3, in which the preganglionic fibres of the sympathetic system arise, you will also find the *rt. & lt. lateral horns*.
- Find the *rt. & lt. ventral roots* and *rt. & lt. dorsal roots*, which form the spinal nerves. The **ventral roots** originate from the ventral <u>and</u> lateral horns (*somatic motor* and *visceral motor*, respectively), whereas the **dorsal roots** enter the dorsal horns. Also find the **dorsal root ganglion** embedded within the dorsal root (a small thickening), which contains the pseudounipolar sensory neurons (both *somatic sensory* and *visceral sensory*). Therefore, the dorsal root ganglion is also called the *spinal sensory ganglion* or short the *spinal ganglion*.
- As mentioned above, the ventral and dorsal roots join to form the **spinal nerve,** which is about 1 cm long and located in the intervertebral foramen. Identify the **four branches** of the spinal nerve:
  (a) *ventral (ant.) ramus* supplying the anterior body wall in a segmental way (e.g. ventral rami of cervical spinal nerves form the cervical & brachial plexus),
  (b) *dorsal (post.) ramus* supplying the posterior body wall in a segmental manner (e.g. dorsal rami of cervical spinal nerves supplying the muscles and skin of the occipital region & posterior neck),
  (c) *ramus communicans* with the *white* and *gray rami communicantes*. The white ramus communicans contains **myelinated preganglionic fibres**, and therefore is only found at spinal cord segments, in which the *visceral motor* lateral horns are present (*sympathetic or parasympathetic*). The fibres in the white ramus run towards the rt. & lt. *paravertebral ganglia* (sympathetic chain) or unpaired *prevertebral ganglia* (e.g. celiac ganglion). **Unmyelinated postganglionic fibres** (e.g. fibres coming back from the paravertebral ganglia) form the gray ramus communicans, which joins the ventral and dorsal rami of the spinal nerves to supply them with visceral motor fibres.
  (d) meningeal ramus running back supplying the meninges.

- Identify the tracts in the white matter: <u>dorsally</u> the *rt. & lt. gracile & cuneate fasciculi*, <u>laterally</u> the *rt. & lt.* lateral corticospinal tract (deep) and *dorsal & ventral spinocerebellar tracts* (superficial), and <u>medially</u> the *lat. spinothalamic & ventral spinothalamic/spinoreticular* tracts, the *vestibulospinal* tract, tectospinal tract and ventral corticospinal tract (fibres that have not crossed in the pyramid).

Per definition, peripheral nerve fibres running *towards* the spinal cord and brainstem are named **afferent** nerve fibres. The neurons of these **sensory** fibres are located in *ganglia* (spinal, cranial nerve & autonomic ganglia). In contrast, peripheral nerve fibres running *from* the spinal cord and brainstem towards the periphery are named **efferent** nerve fibres. The neurons of these **motor** fibres are located in the *spinal cord and brainstem*. **Spinal nerves** have both somatic and visceral components. Therefore, **spinal ganglia** have both *somatic sensory* and *visceral sensory* pseudounipolar neurons (see **Histology***)*. In contrast, **cranial nerve ganglia** contain only neuronal cell types *related to their function* (e.g. the trigeminal ganglion only contains somatic sensory neurones).

Somatic sensory fibres supply the *skin, subcutaneous tissue* and *skeletal muscles*, whereas **visceral sensory** fibres carry sensory information from *superficial* or *deep visceral organs*. **Somatic motor** (and **branchial motor**) fibres innervate skeletal muscles, and **visceral motor** (autonomic) fibres target mainly smooth muscles in visceral organs (e.g. for peristalsis, micturition) and the heart muscle. Postganglionic visceral motor fibres joining the ventral & dorsal rami of spinal nerves supply the sweat glands (*sudomotor*), erector pili muscles (*pilomotor*), wall of blood vessels (*vasomotor*) in the skin, subcutaneous tissue and skeletal muscle.

- **Topographical anatomy of the brainstem including rhomboid fossa**
- Note that he brainstem is composed of the **midbrain** (mesencephalon), the **pons** and the **medulla** (also medulla oblongata). The dorsal brainstem regions are called **tectum** (midbrain), and ventral portions **tegmentum** (midbrain, pons).
- In the **ventral view** of the brainstem, identify the *cerebral peduncles* and *interpeduncular fossa* (midbrain), the *basilar pons* (pons), and the *pyramids* with the *decussation of the pyramidal tract* and *olives* (medulla). Also view the *bulbopontine sulcus & cerebellar angle*, and the *anterior median fissure, rt. & lt. ventrolateral (preolivary)* and *postolivary (retroolivary) sulci*, as these are important <u>landmarks</u> to memorise the exit of cranial nerves out of the brainstem.
- In the **dorsal view**, identify the *four colliculi* (rt. & lt. colliculus sup. and inf.) with their *brachia* (arms), the posterior extension of the *cere<u>bral</u> peduncles* (forms lateral border) and the *trigonum of lateral lemniscus* (acoustic pathways) in the midbrain. Next, find the *sup., middle* and *inf. cere<u>bellar</u> peduncles* around the dorsal pontine region. In the medulla, find the three sulci (*dorsal median, dorsal intermediate & dorsolateral sulci*), the *tubercula gracilis & cuneatus* (formed by respective nuclei at the termination zone of fasciculi gracilis & cuneatus), and *tuberculum cinereum*.

- The **rhomboid fossa** forms the **base of the 4th ventricle** (**dorsal view**). Identify its **borders** by finding the *sup. medullary velum, cerebellar peduncles, lateral recess, inf. medullary velum*, and *obex*. Next view the **base of the fossa** with the *dorsal median sulcus* and *sulcus limitans* dividing the brainstem into vertical columns. Cranial to the *stria medullaris*, find the *colliculus facialis (abducens nucl. with fibres of CN. VII), dentate nucleus of cerebellum* and *sup. fovea*, and caudal to the striae the *hypoglossal trigone, vagal trigone & inf. fovea.*

The **brainstem** does not only harbour the nuclei of the *cranial nerves*, but also regions involved in a *variety of other functions*, e.g. the diffuse, poorly differentiated reticular formation occupies the tegmentum of brainstem. Centres in the **medulla** control eye and head movements, the gag reflex (CN IX, X), swallowing, coughing and vomiting. Other centres regulate heart and respiratory function and visceral activity. The **pons** contains centres important for motor regulation (connection to neocerebellum), lateral eye movements, the corneal blink reflex (CN V, VII), and facial expression and chewing. **Midbrain** centres control vertical eye movements, the pupillary light reflex (CN II, III) and orienting responses (auditory and visual reflexes). The brainstem further regulates arousal and consciousness, and modulates pain.

Many **ascending** and **descending** *sensory and motor fibre systems* originate or terminate in the brainstem or pass through. Therefore, lesions of the brainstem are often a *combination of deficits* including defects in cranial nerve nuclei, sensory & motor tracts, and other functions controlled by specific centres [e.g. *lat. medullary Wallenberg's syndrome* due to an occlusion of the post. inf. cerebellar artery with ipsilat. facial numbness, contralat. pain & temperature loss, cerebellar ataxia, autonomic symptoms, and deficits in nuclei of lower cranial nerves (vestibular nuclei-dizziness; ambiguus-paralysis of soft palate, pharynx & larynx)].

- **Horizontal sections through the brainstem**

- At **mid-olivary level** of the **medulla**, view <u>ventrally</u> the *pyramidal tract* and the *inferior olive*, in the <u>midline</u> the *medial lemniscus* and *medial longitudinal fasciculus*, and <u>dorsally</u> the *hypoglossal nucleus, dorsal motor nucleus of vagus* and *nucleus of solitary tract* (in medial lateral order).

- In a section through the **middle of the pons**, view <u>ventrally</u> *corticospinal & corticopontine fibres* with *pontine nuclei* embedded between the fibres, and <u>at/near the base of the 4th ventricle</u> the *medial lemniscus, lateral lemniscus, central tegmental tract, medial longitudinal fasciculus* and *sup. cerebellar peduncle.*

- In the **midbrain** at the **level of the superior colliculus**, view <u>ventrally</u> the *rt. & lt. cerebral peduncles* with the *interpeduncular fossa*, in the <u>middle</u> the substantia nigra and red nucleus (in lateromed. order), and <u>at/near the base of the 4th ventricle</u> the *oculomotor nucleus* and *central tegmental tract*.

- **Find** the mesencephalic/pontine/caudal raphe nuclei (serotonergic) in the midline, locus coeruleus (dark blue) at the 4th ventricle/near colliculus facialis (noradrenergic) & pedunculopontine nucl. at sup. cerebellar peduncle (cholinergic).

- **Cranial nerve exits in brainstem**
- All **cranial nerve nuclei** are located in the **brainstem** with the **exception** of *olfactory & optic nerves*, but the nuclei of some cranial nerves **extend** into the spinal cord (*trigeminal & accessory nerves*). The *hypoglossal nerve* is a **modified spinal nerve** with somatic motor fibres, which became a cranial nerve due to the fusion of occipital vertebra with the skull bone during development. The cranial nerves are numbered in the order they exit the brainstem. Cranial nerve nuclei are organised in *columns* (*in mediolateral direction*: somatic motor, parasympathetic, branchial motor, visceral sensory, somatic sensory).
- **Ventrally**, view the *oculomotor nerve* (CN. III) exiting the midbrain in the interpeduncular fossa, the *trigeminal nerve* (CN. V) perforating the middle cerebellar peduncle, the abducens nerve (CN. VI) at the bulbopontine sulcus, the facial (CN. VII) & vestibulocochlear nerves (CN. VIII) at the cerebellar angle, the glossopharyngeal (CN. IX), vagus (CN. X) and accessory nerves (CN. XI, cranial & spinal roots) at the postolivary sulcus, and the hypoglossal nerve (CN. XII) at the ventrolateral sulcus. **Dorsally**, identify the *trochlear nerve* (CN. IV).

Cranial nerve	No.	Brainstem nucleus	Type
olfactory	I	n/a (respiratory mucosa)	special sensory (smell)
optic	II	n/a (retinal ganglion cells)	special sensory (visual)
oculomotor	III	oculomotor	somatic motor
	III	Edinger-Westphal	parasympathetic
trochlear	IV	trochlear	somatic motor
trigeminal	V	main sensory, spinal	somatic sensory
	V	mesencephalic	branchial motor (masticatory)
abducens	VI	abducens	somatic motor
facial	VII	facial	branchial motor (facial expression)
	VII	superior salivatory	parasympathetic
	VII	nucleus of solitary tract	visceral sensory & gustatory
vestibulocochlear	VIII	cochlear (two nuclei)	special sensory (acoustic)
	VIII		special sensory (balance)
glossopharyngeal	IX	ambiguus	branchial motor
		inferior salivatory	parasympathetic
		nucleus of solitary tract	visceral sensory & gustatory
vagus	X	ambiguus	branchial motor
		dorsal motor	parasympathetic
		nucleus of solitary tract	visceral sensory & gustatory
accessory	XI	ambiguus	branchial motor
	XI	spinal accessory (C1-5)	branchial motor
hypoglossal	XI	hypoglossal	somatic motor

- **Organisation of the cerebellum**
- Note that the cerebellum is located in the posterior cranial fossa below the cerebellar tent (tentorium cerebelli). It has two **hemispheres** and a **vermis** in the middle. In the **superior view**, identify the *sup. vermis* (with the *central lobule, culmen, declive, folium*), and in the hemispheres the *ant. & post. lobes* separated by the *primary fissure*. On the **inferior surface**, find the *inf. vermis* (with the *nodule, uvula, pyramid, tuber*), extension of the *sup. vermis* (with the *central lobule, lingula*), and the *post. lobes*.
- In a **median sagittal section** through the cerebellum, you can identify the *parts of the vermis* separated by fissures in the following order: *lingula, central lobule, culmen, declive, folium, tuber, pyramid, uvula*, and *nodule*.
- In a **tilted horizontal cut** through the cerebellum from the sup. cerebellar peduncle to the nodule you can see the *cerebellar nuclei* (from lateral to medial the *dentate, emboliform, globose & fastigial nuclei*) and the *decussation of sup. cerebellar peduncles*.

The cerebellum can be divided into an **archicerebellum, paleocerebellum**, and **neocerebellum**. The archicerebellar **floccular nodular lobe**, attributed to the *vestibulocerebellum* and intensely interconnected with the vestibular nuclei, is important for balance, and eye and head movements. The paleocerebellar **anterior lobe** belonging to the *spinocerebellum* is the termination zone of the *ant. and post. spinocerebellar tracts* relaying somatic sensory information to the cerebellum for the regulation of muscle tone and walking. The neocerebellar **posterior lobe** assigned to the *pontocerebellum* receives afferents from the contralateral motor cortex through the cortico-ponto-cerebellar tract (synapse in pons) for the coordination of fine & skilled movements, and also for cognition.

The **cerebellar cortex** has *three layers* - the granular cell layer, Purkinje cell layer and molecular layer. Cerebellar afferent are called *mossy fibres* (from regions connected specifically to *vestibulo-, spino-, and pontocerebellum*) terminating in the granule cell layer, and *climbing fibres* from the *inferior olive* synapsing with dendrites of Purkinje cells in the molecular layer. Purkinje cells are inhibitory neurons controlling the output of the cerebellar nuclei. In turn, the cerebellar nuclei provide feedback projections to the reticular formation/vestibular nuclei giving rise to the **reticulo- and vestibulospinal tracts** (*fastigial nucleus from vestibulocerebellum*), to the red nucleus giving rise to the **rubrospinal tract** (*emboliform & globose nuclei from spinocerebellum*), and the ventral lateral thalamus giving rise to thalamocortical projections (*dentate nucleus from pontocerebellum*).

- **Meninges and attachments of cranial nerves**
- View the outermost **dura mater** (dense membrane adhering to the skull inside) with its external (parietal) and internal (visceral) layers, and the **arachnoid membrane** coursing directly below the dura mater (without adhering to it). The

arachnoid membrane sends out *arachnoid trabeculae* that are attached to the innermost layer called **pia mater** that follows the contours of the brain surface.

- Identify the **epidural space** between the skull bone and dura mater, the **subdural space** between the dura mater and arachnoid membrane, and the **subarachnoid space** between the arachnoid membrane and pia mater.
- View the **venous sinuses** running *between* the parietal & visceral layers of the dura mater (*sup. & inf. sagittal, cavernous, sup. & inf. petrosal, straight* and *transverse* sinus; internal jugular vein is continuation of sigmoid sinus).
- Examine the dural extensions formed by two visceral layers of the dura mater: the **falx cerebri** separating the two cerebral hemispheres, the **tentorium cerebelli** separating the occipital lobe from the posterior cranial fossa.
- View the attachments of **cranial nerves passing** through the **dura mater** on the skull base (sup. aspect) heading toward the *sup. orbital fissure* [CN. III running most superiorly lat. to post. clinoid process; CN. IV & CN. V$_1$ coursing over the free edge of the petrosal bone (petrous part of temporal bone); and CN. VI perforating the dura mater at the clivus], entering the *internal acoustic meatus* (CN. VII an VIII), passing through the *jugular foramen* (CN. IX, X and XI) and running through the *hypoglossal canal* (CN. XII).
- After **removal of the dura mater** (on one side of middle cranial fossa only), view the cranial nerves running through the *sup. orbital fissure* (CN. III, IV, V$_1$ and VI) and the *trigeminal ganglion* with the three branches of the trigeminal nerve (CN. V$_1$, V$_2$ and V$_3$) leaving the intracranial cavity.

*P.S.: For **bleedings** in the epidural, subdural and subarachnoid spaces, and further details see **Skull-I and II practical sessions**.*

- **Blood supply of the brain and spinal cord**
- Revise the **extracranial course** of **major arteries supplying the brain**:

(a) *rt. & lt. internal carotid artery* (branch of common carotid artery) coursing through the carotid canal (**anterior circuit**), and

(b) *rt. & lt. vertebral artery* (branch of subclavian artery) coursing in the transverse cervical foramina and entering the intracranial cavity though the foramen magnum (**posterior circuit**).

- Now examine the **intracranial course** of **major arteries supplying the brain**:

(a) **rt. & lt. internal carotid arteries** running at the *lateral border of the sella turcica* (hypophyseal groove) through the cavernous sinus in a *sigmoid-shaped* curve. On either side, the internal carotid artery gives rise to the *sup. & inf. hypophyseal, hypothalamic, anterolat. central (lenticulostriate)* and *ophthalmic arteries* before it contributes to the circle of Willis.

(b) **rt. & lt. vertebral arteries** giving off two branches forming the unpaired *ant. spinal artery* as well as the paired *PICAs* (post. inf. cerebellar arteries) **before** they join to form the basilar artery. The **basilar artery** gives rise to the paired *AICA* (post. inf. cerebellar artery), *pontine & mesencephalic arteries* and *sup. cerebellar artery* as well as to a few *posteromedial (paramedian) central arteries*, before it divides into the *rt. & lt. post. cerebral arteries* (end branches).

- Study the **cerebral arterial circle (Willis)**, or short the *circle of Willis*, securing the blood supply of the brain through anastomoses of major arteries coming bilaterally from the ant. & post. circuits. The circle is formed at the *base of the brain* by the underlined ant. communicating artery, and the underlined *ant. cerebral, internal carotid, post. communicating*, and *post. cerebral arteries*. Also view the short branches (bilat.) of the *circle of Willis* called **perforating arteries:** *Posteromedial perforating arteries* supplying mainly thalamic regions (from P1 segments of post. cerebral arteries incorporated into the circle & post. communicating arteries), the *sup. & inf. hypophyseal, hypothalamic & lenticulostriate arteries* (from intracranial segment of internal carotid artery) and anteromedial perforating arteries supplying mainly the ant. basal forebrain (from A1 segment of ant. cerebral artery & two ant. communicating arteries).
- Inspect the **cerebral regions** directly supplied by the paired **cerebral arteries:**

  (a) *ant. cerebral artery* and its branches [*recurrent artery of Heubner* to dorsomedial striatum, and the *med. orbitofrontal, frontopolar, callosomarginal* and *pericallosal* arteries with the *precuneal* artery (end branch)];

  (b) *middle cerebral artery* with its deep branches (*ant. choroidal artery* and *lenticulostriate perforating arteries*), and cortical branches - the *sup. trunk* [*lat. orbitofrontal, prefrontal, precentral & central (Rolandic)* branches] and *inf. trunk* [*ant., middle & post. temporal, ant./ post. parietal* and *angular* branches];

  (c) *post. cerebral artery* with its deep (*perforating, choroidal*) and cortical branches (*ant.& post. temporal* and *med. occipital arteries*, latter dividing into the *parietooccipital & calcarine branches*).
- Study the **superficial cerebral veins** coursing together with the arteries & the *inf. anastomotic vein* (*Labbé*), **bridging veins** (drain into sup. sagittal sinus) and **deep veins** [paired *basal* (Rosenthal) & *internal cerebral veins* draining into the unpaired *great cerebral vein* (Galen), which then drains into the *straight sinus.*
- View the blood supply to the **spinal cord** by the underlined ant. *spinal artery/vein* and underlined *post. spinal artery/vein* (upper portions of ant. spinal artery from vertebral artery, rest coming from/draining into segmental vessels).

An *occlusion of a cerebral* artery leads to an **ischaemic brain infarction**, usually resulting from arteriosclerosis (e.g. by *thrombus* formation) or *embolism*. A **haemorrhagic brain infarction** is induced by an intracranial bleeding. Causes are rupturing blood vessels [e.g. in hypertension, vascular malformations (arterio-venous, cavernous), tumours or subarachnoid bleeds perforating into the brain], venous thrombosis (blockade of blood flow) or contusions (e.g. traumatic).

The **circle of Willis** is subject to *high interindividual variation*, which has a big impact on its capacity to compensate an occlusion of a major artery. **Lenticulostriate arteries** (perforating arteries) supply large portions of the *basal ganglia & internal capsule* with devastating effects in case of an occlusion. Occlusions of the **middle cerebral artery** results in a hemiparesis affecting the upper limb more than the lower limb, whereas the leg is more severely paralysed if the **ant. cerebral artery** is affected. Occlusion of the **post. cerebral artery** leads to contralat. homonymous hemianopia (& deficits in cognitive functions).

19. NEUROANATOMY - II

In this session, we will study the **ventricular system, coronal sections** through the **cerebral hemispheres** and **diencephalic regions**.

19.1 DISSECTIONS

- **Dissection of lateral ventricles**

The **purpose** of this dissection is to see the *ant.* (*frontal*), *post.* (*occipital*) and *inf.* (*temporal*) <u>*horns of the lateral ventricle*</u> connected by its *central part*.

- First, make a **<u>transversal (tilted) cut</u>** through the cerebral hemispheres in the **plane** that runs **parallel to the inferior border** of the *trunk of the corpus callosum* (plane above *genu & splenium of corpus callosum*). Now you can see the *rt. & lt. frontal & occipital horns* and *central parts* of the *lateral ventricles.*

- In order to **dissect** the *temporal horn* of the *lateral ventricle*, **<u>identify</u>** the *middle temporal gyrus* (*rt. or lt.*), and carefully **<u>dissect it out</u>** until you **reach** the temporal horn of the lateral ventricle **at one point**. Hereby, try to keep the dissection in the plane running parallel to the basis of the temporal lobe. Once you have found the ventricle, gently **remove the whole** middle temporal gyrus by following the course of the temporal horn (be careful not to break the tissue).

19.2 PROSECTIONS AND MODELS

- **Ventricles and their connections**

- There are **four ventricles** in the brain, all lined with ependyma. View the 1st and 2nd ventricles (*lateral ventricles*) surrounded mainly by the telencephalon (except at the lamina affixa), the *3rd ventricle* surrounded by the diencephalon, and the *4th ventricle* embedded within the metencephalon.

- View the connections *between the ventricles* as well as between the 4th ventricle and *cisterns* (*subarachnoid space*): The lateral ventricles and the 3rd ventricle are connected through the *interventricular foramina* (Monro); the 3rd and 4th ventricles through the *cerebral aqueduct,* and the 4th ventricle and cerebellomedullary cistern through one *median aperture* (Magendie) and two *lateral apertures* (Luschka). Here, the choroid plexus extends from the 4th ventricle into the subarachnoid space forming the "flower basket of Bochdalek".

- Part of the choroid plexus of the fourth ventricle protruding through Luschka's foramen.

- The extension of the most caudal ventricle (the 4th ventricle) is the spinal canal, which is located centrally within the spinal cord.

- View the **arachnoid villi** or **granulations** (*Pacchionian bodies*) extending into the sup. sagittal sinus (venous sinus) at the vertex of the brain.

- Examine the **<u>lateral ventricles</u>** (paired) using the dissection prepared above:

(a) **Frontal horn** reaching forward from the *column of fornix* at the *ant. border of interventricular foramen* (post. border). Anteriorly it is bound by the *genu & rostrum of corpus callosum*, medially by the *septum pellucidum*, ventrally & laterally by the *head (caput) of caudate nucl.* extending into the lateral ventricle, and dorsally by the *trunk of corpus callosum.*

(b) **Central part** stretching from the *interventricular foramen* (ant. border) to the *splenium of corpus callosum* (post. border). Find dorsally the *trunk of corpus callosum*, medially the *septum pellucidum & fornix* (corpus), and ventrolaterally the *head of caudate nucl.*, which thins out in anteroposterior direction and becomes the *body (corpus)*. The *body of caudate nucl.* extends medially to the *groove* that is interposed between the caudate nucl. and *thalamus*, and harbours the *stria terminalis & sup. thalamostriate vein.* Here identify the **lamina affixa** (in lat. ventricle, but lines thalamus) reaching from this groove up to the attachment of the *choroid plexus* at the *taenia choroidea.* Now view medial to the choroid plexus at the posteromedial corner of the central part, the *hippocampus* (near trigone of lat. ventricle/splenium of corpus callosum) & *fornix* (crus), and follow the course of these structures (incl. choroid plexus) to the temporal horn.

(c) **Occipital horn** reaching backward from the corpus callosum with *collateral trigone* (lat.), *calcar avis* (med.) inferiorly and the posterior tip (post.).

(d) In the **temporal horn**, view the course of structures extending to the central part of the ventricle. Find medially the *choroid plexus*, laterally white matter (inf. longitudinal fasciculus, post. limb of ant. commissure), ventrally the *hippocampus* (including pes) with the *fornix/fimbria hippocampi* & collateral eminence (formed by collateral sulcus, reaches to collateral trigone), dorsally at ventricle roof the *tail (cauda) of caudate nucleus* running together with stria terminalis, and anteriorly the *amygdaloid body.*

- In the **3rd ventricle**, identify anteriorly the *lamina terminalis, ant. commissure & supraoptic recess* (above optic chiasm), dorsally the *interventricular foramen, tela choroidea & choroid plexus* of the 3rd ventricle and the *fornix*, posteriorly the *cuneus, suprapineal recess* (between *habenular commissure* & pineal body), *pineal recess* (between pineal body & *post. commissure*) and *cerebral aqueduct*, and ventrally the *infundibular recess, hypothalamic nuclei* (e.g. mammillary bodies) reaching to the roof of the mesencephalon in the midline posteriorly. The wall of the 3rd ventricle is formed laterally by the hypothalamus and thalamus (periventricular nuclei) separated by the hypothalamic sulcus, and can be interrupted in the middle by the interthalamic adhaesion.

- In the **4th ventricle**, we have already examined the *rhomboid fossa* forming the anterior border (see **Brainstem** in **Neuroanatomy-I tutorial**). Now view superiorly & inferiorly the two connections of the ventricle, which are the *cerebral aqueduct* and *central spinal canal*, respectively. Posteriorly, the 4th ventricle is bound by the *sup. & inf. medullary velum* (latter reaches obex), *fastigium* (extends into cerebellum) and *median aperture* (Magendie). The ventricle wall is formed laterally by the *cerebellar peduncles, inf. medullary velum* & the *lateral recesses* extending up to the *lateral apertures* (Luschka). At the inf. medullary velum, find also the *tela choroidea* for the attachment of the *choroid plexus of the 4th ventricle.*

The ventricles are lined by **ependyma**, a selectively permeable thin epithelial layer. **Cerebrospinal fluid** (CSF) is secreted into each ventricle by its own **choroid plexus**. In healthy individuals, it is a clear water-like liquid, its contents clearly differing from blood, which is ensured by the **blood-CSF-barrier**. It provides also the extracellular fluid in the neuropil, and therefore corresponds to the *lymph of the brain*. The CSF **circulates** from the lateral ventricles to the 3rd, and from there to the 4th ventricle. Finally, it enters the subarachnoid space through the med. & lat. apertures, and flows toward the **arachnoid villi** around the sup. sagittal sinus, where it is absorbed. The arachnoid villi have a filter and barrier function for draining the CSF from the subarachnoid space back into the venous system, and the amount drained depends on the intracranial pressure. The **thecal sacs** (dura and arachnoid mater) around the *roots of cranial and spinal nerves* are the second site of CSF absorption.

Disturbances in the **circulation** of CSF can lead to congestion with enlargement of the ventricular system called **hydrocephalus**. An *internal hydrocephalus* occurs (congestion of ventricles only) if the circulation is disrupted before the CSF reaches the subarachnoid space. It is usually induced by an obstruction of ventricular connections (e.g. by a tumour). In a *communicating hydrocephalus*, both the ventricles <u>and</u> subarachnoid space are enlarged. Common reasons are an excess of CSF production, disturbances in CSF resorption (e.g. after meningitis) or a secondary communicating hydrocephalus resulting from brain atrophy.

Circumventricular organs are regions located in the midline at or near the 3rd and 4th ventricle (subfornical organ, median eminence of hypothalamus, subcommissural organ, pineal gland and area postrema). Since they have no blood-brain barrier, they are the site for chemosensation, diffusion of molecules, and neuroendocrine secretion (see hypothalamus).

- **Coronal (frontal) sections of the cerebral hemispheres**

These can be viewed in *wet specimens*, *plastinated sections* or *histological sections* of the brain (latter usually Weigert stain for myelin). As a **reference point** for coronal levels, the plane running through the **ant. commissure** was used [see http://www.thehumanbrain.info/; Atlas of the Human Brain by Mai, Paxinos & Voss, 2007, Elsevier, San Diego). Please note that some structures are quite small and may not be hit exactly at the coordinates provided due to minor changes in the sectioning angle. Differences can also be expected between wet specimens versus plastinated/histological sections (shrinkage), and there are considerable interindividual differences in the size of brains and ventricles (age-/sex-related).

Level I) In a coronal section through the frontal lobe (approx. at <u>-10 mm</u> or 1 cm rostral to ant. commissure; temporal pole lose & usually missing), the *corpus callosum, frontal horn of lat. ventricle*, and *internal capsule* can be seen. The internal capsule separates the *head of caudate nucl.* and *putamen* only incomplete-ly (latter two regions <u>dorsal striatum</u>), whereas the ventral/linked parts are called *accumbens nucleus* and *fundus of striatum* (<u>ventral striatum</u>). The *claustrum* is separated from the putamen by the *external capsule* & from the insula by the *extreme capsule*. Also identify <u>cortical areas</u> in the *cingulate gyrus* (dors. to corpus callosum), *insula* and *frontal lobe* (sup., middle & inf. frontal gyri and frontal operculum, piriform cortex, straight gyrus and subcallosal area). If the *temporal* lobe is available at this level, view cortical areas described at Level II.

Level II) At <u>0 mm</u> (level of ant. commissure), identify <u>below the corpus callosum</u> the *septum* (septum pellucidum*, med. & lat. septal nuclei, column of fornix), bed nucl. of stria terminalis* and *head of caudate nucl.* (all three structures at the *frontal horn of lat. ventricle*), the *internal capsule, putamen and external & internal pallidum* (latter three often summarised as lentiform nucleus), *external capsule, claustrum, extreme capsule, ant. commissure* and *optic chiasm*. <u>Cortical regions</u> hit at this level are *limbic* (cingulate gyrus), *frontal* (sup. frontal, middle frontal & precentral gyri and frontal operculum), *insular* and *temporal areas* (planum polare, sup., middle & inf. temporal gyri and fusiform, perirhinal & parahippocampal gyri).

Level III) At approx. <u>+5 mm</u> (post. to ant. commissure), view the same areas mentioned above except the ant. commissure, optic chiasm & head of caudate nucl., which are now replaced by the *post. limb of ant. commissure & optic tract* (located more laterally) and *body of caudate nucl.* Also identify the *interventricular foramina* (Monro), *3rd ventricle* surrounded by the *thalamus* and *hypothalamus,* and the *amygdaloid body* in the <u>temporal lobe</u>. Embedded within the hypothalamus find the *fornix*. Next view the <u>cortical areas</u> in the *insula*, and *limbic* (cingulate gyrus), *frontal* (ant. paracentral, sup. frontal, middle frontal & precentral gyri and frontal operculum) and *temporal lobes* (planum polare, ant. transverse gyrus, sup., middle & inf. temporal gyri and fusiform, perirhinal & parahippocampal gyri).

Level IV) At approx. <u>+10 to +15 mm</u>, the picture is quite similar to Level III except that striatopallidal areas become smaller, whereas the thalamus occupies a large territory, and the *ant. commissure/interventricular foramen* cannot be seen anymore. The *optic tract* may join the internal capsule (included to the capsule by some authors). <u>Below the thalamus</u> identify the *mammilothalamic tract, subthalamic nucleus & mammillary body* (part of hypothalamus), and in the <u>temporal lobe</u> the *uncus of hippocampus* and *tail of the caudate nucl.* at the *roof* of the *temporal horn of lat. ventricle*. Also identify <u>other cortical areas</u> including the *cingulate gyrus, insula*, and areas in the *frontal* (ant. paracentral & precentral gyri, very short sector of frontal operculum), *temporal* (planum polare, ant. transverse gyrus, planum temporale; sup., middle & inf. temporal gyri; and fusiform, perirhinal & parahippocampal gyri) and *parietal lobes* (if present small areas of postcentral gyrus & parietal operculum).

Level V) At approx. <u>+22 to +25 mm</u>, view around <u>the lat. ventricle</u> (central part) the *body (corpus) of fornix, corpus callosum/white matter, body of caudate nucl.*, and the *lamina affixa*. The lamina affixa stretches from the groove containing the *stria terminalis* & *sup. thalamostriate vein* (medial border of caudate nucl.) to the *attachment of choroid plexus* at the *ventricular surface of thalamus*.

<u>Below the lat. ventricle</u>, identify the *subarachnoid space* (velum interpositum) containing the *pineal gland* (at coronal levels +25 to 30 mm), the diencephalic *thalamus* and *med. & lat. geniculate body* (the latter two metathalamus, for

acoustic and visual pathways, respectively), *3rd or 4th ventricle* (depending on sectioning plane), and the mesencephalic *red nucleus, substantia nigra & cerebral peduncles* (latter may or may not have lost its continuation with internal capsule). In the temporal lobe focus first on the *temporal horn* of the *lat. ventricle* that is surrounded by the *choroid plexus* (medially), *white matter & stria terminalis* (dorsally), *tail of caudate nucl.* (dorsolaterally), and hippocampus (ventrally). Note that the lat. geniculate body has the shape of a striped hat at this level (layers receiving separate input from the two eyes), at which the hippocampal formation is classically studied (e.g. in neuropathological examination). In the hippocampal formation, identify the *dentate gyrus* and *hippocampal* (hilus, CA1-3) *& subicular sectors*. The *parahippocampal gyrus* is located inf. to the hippocampus and separated from the adjacent *fusiform gyrus* by the *collateral sulcus*. Next find the sup. temporal surface with the ant. & post. transverse gyri (Heschl's gyri containing the primary auditory cortex), and laterally the sup., middle & inf. temporal gyri. Other cortical regions are the *cingulate gyrus, insula*, and areas in the *frontal* (ant. paracentral & precentral gyri) and *parietal lobes* (postcentral gyri, parietal operculum).

Level VI) The coronal level at approx. +30 mm is best for finding the *pineal gland* if it is preserved in the specimen (see also Level V). In the thalamus, the pulvinar occupies the largest part except the mediodorsal thalamic nucleus. In the brainstem, the cerebral aqueduct, periaqueductal gray and pretectal area can be seen in the midbrain, but pontine regions may also be present. In the cortex find the *cingulate gyrus*, and *frontal* (ant. paracentral & precentral gyri), *parietal* (postcentral & supramarginal gyri, parietal operculum) and *temporal regions* [on sup. temporal surface the transverse temporal gyri & planum temporale; laterally sup., middle & inf. temporal gyri; ventromedially fusiform & post. parahippocampal gyri].

Level VII) At approx. +40 to +45 mm, the posterior tip of the central part of the lat. ventricle reaching to the occipital horn can be seen. At the medial border of the ventricle, inspect the *splenium of corpus callosum & post. hippocampus* (preserved in amygdalahippocampectomy in intractable epilepsy). Other cortical areas are the *cingulate gyrus*, and *parietal* (precuneus, post. paracentral, postcentral & supramarginal gyri) *& temporal areas* (laterally sup., middle & inf. temporal gyri; ventromedially fusiform, lingual & post. parahippocampal gyri).

Level VIII) At approx. +50 to +53 mm, view the *ant. calcarine sulcus* and its protrusion into the occipital horn of the lat. ventricle called *calcar avis*, which is formed by fibres of the optic radiation. You can also identify the post. extension of the *cingulate gyrus*, and several *parietal* (precuneus, sup. parietal lobe, supramarginal gyrus), *temporal* (laterally sup., middle & inf. temporal gyri, medially fusiform & lingual gyri) and *occipital cortical areas* (region around ant. calcarine sulcus).

Level IX) At approx. +65 to 80 mm, view the *calcarine sulcus* now extending deeply into the med. occipital lobe, and find the *primary visual cortex* at the sulcus (Brodmann area A17 or striate cortex) easily identifiable by the Gennari stripe (in cortical layer four). Note that the A17 is found around the full extent of the calcarine gyrus up to the occipital pole (at approx. +100 mm). Further areas in the *occipital lobe* are the A18 (secondary visual cortex encircling A17) & other occipital gyri (located mostly inferiorly), in the temporal lobe the middle & inf. temporal gyri (posteriorly also temporooccipital transition zone), and in the *parietal lobe* the parietooccipital transition zone & precuneus (both regions dors. to parietooccipital sulcus) as well as the angular gyrus.

- **Diencephalic regions**

In the coronal sections above, we have grossly identified the *hypothalamus*, and *thalamus*, and mentioned regions in the *subthalamus* and *metathalamus*. Now we will have a closer look at these structures in the region around the *3rd ventricle*, and the *pituitary gland* (*hypophysis*) and *epithalamus*.

Hypothalamus and pituitary gland

The **hypothalamus** can be seen best at mid-hypothalamic level (Level III above, at +5 mm), where it has the shape of a triangle with the fornix in the middle. However, in reality it extends from about the level of the ant. commissure & optic chiasm (at 0 mm) to the end of mammillary bodies (at approx. +12 to +13 mm).

- Directly above the optic chiasm find the suprachiasmatic nucl. (involved in regulation of circadian rhythms). The region between the ant. commissure & optic chiasm contains the *periventricular, paraventricular & medial preoptic* nuclei and the *lateral hypothalamic* area.
- At approx. +2 or +3 mm, view between the fornix & basis of hypothalamus the *paraventricular nucl.*, the *dors. & lat. hypothalamic areas*, and the *ventromed. hypothalamic, infundibular* (tuberal) and *supraoptic nucl.* (above optic tract). Also find the *medial eminence* at the *tuber cinereum* (no blood-brain-barrier).
- At mid-hypothalamic level (+5 mm) find medial to the fornix the *peri- & paraventricular, dorsomed. hypothalamic*, and *infundibular (tuberal)* nuclei. The region lateral to the fornix contains the *lat. hypothalamic area, lat. tuberal nucl. tuberomammillary* (histaminergic cell group) & *supraoptic nuclei*.
- At post. levels (+10 to +12 mm) identify the *mammillary bodies*, and *post. & lat. hypothalamic areas* (med. & lat. to mammilo-tegmental tract, respectively).
- The **pituitary gland (hypophysis)** is a gland located in the hypophyseal groove. The hypophyseal groove is not only lined ventrally, but also covered dorsally by *dural mater* (diaphragma sellae). The pituitary gland is connected to the hypothalamus through the *infundibular stem* (pituitary stalk; ruptures usually when brain is removed), and therefore may be missing in your specimen.

The hypothalamus is a centre regulating **sympathetic & parasympathetic functions** (e.g. parvicellular paraventricular nucl., lat. hypothalamic area), **endocrine secretion** (magnocellular paraventricular/supraoptic and parvicellular tuberal nuclei), **arousal** (histaminergic tuberomammillary nucl.) and numerous **behaviours** like **feeding** (e.g. ventromedial nucl.) and **sexual behaviour** (e.g. preoptic region). The suprachiasmatic nucl. receives direct input from the retina and is involved in the control **circadian rhythms**.

The paraventricular & supraoptic nuclei you could view in today's tutorial have magnocellular neurons often shown in schematic diagrams of the hypothalamus. These neurons project to the **post. lobe** of the **pituitary gland**, and secrete the hormones vasopressin (also antidiuretic hormone, ADH) and oxytocin there into the blood stream. This is called **neuroendocrine secretion**, because the secretion is carried out by axons and there is no blood-brain-barrier at the site of hormone secretion. The **ant. lobe** of the pituitary gland (derivative of **Rathke's pouch** in the pharynx) secretes hormones regulating energy balance (TSH, ACTH), growth (GH), sexual functions (LH, FSH), milk production (prolactin) and melanocyte activity (MSH). In addition, the **mammillary bodies** in the post. thalamus project to the ant. thalamic nuclei (mammillo-thalamic tract), and are as part of the limbic *Papez-circuit* important for **learning and memory**.

Thalamus, subthalamus and metathalamus

- The **thalamus** is much larger than the hypothalamus reaching approx. from coronal level +5 mm to +35 mm.
- Anterior thalamic regions can be studied well at approx. +10 mm (level of mid-hypothalamus or mammillary bodies depending on sectioning plane). First identify the *internal & external medullary laminae of thalamus* (the latter near the medial border of internal capsule). Medial to the internal medullary lamina find the *paraventricular thalamic nucl.* (midline thalamic nucl. connected to limbic-prefrontal regions & involved in **arousal**) and *ant. thalamic nucl.* (see **Papez-circuit** in **Neuroanatomy – III**). Between the internal & external medullary laminae identify the *ventral ant. nucl.* (relay station in **cortical-dorsal striato-pallidal motor circuits**), and lat. to the external lamina the *reticular thalamic nucl.* (inhibits thalamic relay nuclei, important in **rhythm generation**). Below the thalamic complex view the *zona incerta*, a **subthalamic region** interposed between the thalamus and lateral hypothalamus.
- Mid-thalamic regions can be studied well at approx. +13 mm to +17 mm. The *paraventricular thalamic nucl.* is located most medially (around the 3rd ventricle). The now less prominent internal medullary lamina forms the lat. border of the *mediodorsal thalamic nucl.* (relay station in **limbic-ventr. striato-pallidal-prefrontal pathways**) and separates it from the *ventr. ant. thalamic nucl.* (intermediate location). More laterally find the *ventr. lateral thalamic nucl.* with its ant. and post. subnuclei (often abbreviated as VLA and VLP in textbooks, relay stations in **cortico-dors. striato-pallidal & cortico-ponto-cerebellar circuits**, respectively). The external medullary lamina is seen bet-ween the latter nucl. and the crescent-shaped *reticular thalamic nucl.* (lateral-most location). On its way to the *ant. thalamic nucl.* (located dorsal to medio-dors. nucl.), the mammillo-thalamic tract may split the ventr. ant. thalamic nucl. into med. & lat. halves. The mammillo-tegmental tract (if present at level stu-died) separates the thalamus from the *subthalamic nucl.* (**subthalamic region**, but functionally integrated in basal ganglia circuits) & lat. hypothalamic area.
- At more post. thalamic levels (approx. +22 mm to +25mm), the *reuniens nucl.* appears ventral to the *paraventricular nucl.* (both midline thalamic nucl.). The nucleus dorsal to the *mediodorsal thalamic nucl.* is the *lat. dors. thalamic nucl.*

(replaces ant. thalamic nucl.), whereas nuclei <u>ventral to it</u> are the *parafascicular & centromedian nuclei* (intralaminar thalamic nuclei, **project to striatum**). Furthermore, the ventr. ant. thalamic nucl. disappears, and its territory is occupied first by the *ventr. lat. thalamic nucl.* (see above), and <u>lateral to it</u>, by the *ventr. post. thalamic nucl.* (relay station for **general sensation & taste;** *posterolat. & posteromed. subnuclei*). More posteriorly, however, the *pulvinar nuclei* (particularly **large in primates**), and lateral to them, the *ventr. post. thalamic nucl.* can be seen <u>between the internal & external medullary laminae</u>. View also the *medial & lateral geniculate bodies* (**metathalamic regions**), which are relay stations for the acoustic and visual pathways, respectively (see **Level V** at approx. +22 to +25 mm in coronal sections above).
- The <u>caudal end of the thalamus</u> (levels +30 to +35 mm) contains the *pulvinar*.

The **thalamus** is regarded as the **gate of conscious perception**, because it is integrated into many neuronal loops/circuits and ascending fibre systems, whereas its **main target is the cerebral cortex** (except reticular thalamic nucl.).

The **specific or relay thalamic nuclei** are stations for **sensory & motor pathways** (except for olfactory afferents):
- for *visual* pathways the lat. geniculate body,
- for *auditory* pathways the med. geniculate body,
- for *somatosensory* (*lat. spino-thalamic & post. column*) pathways the ventr. posterolat. thalamic nucl. (usually abbreviated as VPL),
- for ***trigemino-thalamic somatosensory*** pathways the ventr. posteromed. thalamic nucl. (usually abbreviated as VPM),
- for *taste* pathways the ventr. posteromed. thalamic nucl. (VPM)
- for *cerebellar feedback* to motor cortical areas the ventr. lat. thalamic nucl. (abbreviated as VL),
- for *feedback from basal ganglia* to motor cortical areas the ventr. ant. thalamic nucl. (abbreviated as VA), and part of the VL.

The **thalamic association nuclei** receive considerable input from the cerebral cortex and reciprocate these projections (mediodorsal nucl. limbic-prefrontal pathways important in *motivation*, ant. thalamic nuclei Papez circuit for *learning & memory*, pulvinar connected to *widespread association cortical areas*).

The **non-specific thalamic nuclei** can be divided in nuclei involved in functions such as *arousal* that are connected *widely to cortical-limbic* (midline nuclei, e.g. paraventricular, reuniens) or *cortical-striatal areas*, (intralaminar nuclei, e.g. parafascicular & centromedian nuclei); and the reticular thalamic nucl. *inhibiting other thalamic nuclei*, important in *rhythm generation* and *generalised epilepsy* (receives widespread cortical input but does not project to cerebral cortex).

Epithalamus including pineal gland
The *habenular nuclei* occupy a small region at the transition between the di- & mesencephalon that can be seen best in the *habenular trigone* (at the wall of the 3rd ventricle). The **pineal gland (epiphysis)**, often missing in specimens, produces *melatonin* important in the regulation of **circadian rhythms**.

20. NEUROANATOMY -III

Today we will study the **telencephalon**, its relationship to the **basal ganglia** & the **cerebral white matter**.

20.1 DISSECTIONS

- **Dissection of tracts in cerebral white matter**

Dissection can be easier if fixed brains are kept frozen at -20°, and thawed before the practical session. Use a tweezers to dissect bluntly (do not cut with a scalpel).

- One aim is the dissection of **cortical commissural fibres** (radiatio of corpus callosum), **cingulum, forceps minor** (anteriorly), **forceps major** (posteriorly) & **tapetum** (post.-ventrally).To achieve this take one cerebral hemisphere and carefully remove the gray matter of all supracallosal gyri (sup. frontal, paracentral & cingulate gyri, precuneus & cuneus), and reveal the fibre tracts.

- A second aim is the dissection of the <u>**external capsule**</u> as well as the **cortico-spinal/cortico-nuclear** (also cortico-bulbar), **cortico-pontine** & **cortico-thala-mic fibres** running in the <u>**internal capsule**</u>. For this purpose, turn the hemisphere and dissect from laterally. To <u>find the *external capsule*</u>, you must first remove cortical gyri (e.g. opercula) to approach the insula, and then remove the extreme capsule/insula. Now leave a square-shaped region of the external capsule and carry on deeper dissection to <u>find the *internal capsule*</u>. For revealing the *internal capsule*, you must remove the external capsule and lentiform nucl. (putamen, external & internal pallidum). Note that once you have arrived at the internal capsule and see the *cortico-spinal/cortico-nuclear/cortico-pontine fibres*, you must cut out a window from these fibre tracts to see the deeper (more medially) coursing *cortico-thalamic fibres.*

20.2 PROSECTIONS AND MODELS

- **Overview of telencephalon (lat. view)**
- First find the <u>central & lateral (Sylvian) sulci</u>. The central sulcus separates the **frontal lobe** from the **parietal lobe**, and the lateral sulcus the frontal & parietal lobes from the **temporal lobe**. Next find the <u>preoccipital incisure</u>, which marks the inf. point of the dorsoventral line that separates the parietal & temporal lobes from the **occipital lobe**.

- <u>On the frontal lobe</u> view the *sup., middle & inf. frontal gyri,* which are three gyri running horizontally, but may not be separated completely by sulci. Anterior to the <u>central sulcus</u> find the *precentral gyrus* containing the **primary motor cortex**. Discuss the location of areas on the gyrus controlling movements of the lower limb, trunk, upper limb (especially hand & thumb), face, larynx & tongue in dorso-ventral direction (according to *motor homunculus*). Now find the sulcus coursing ant. to the precentral gyrus, the <u>precentral sulcus</u>, and the *pre-precentral gyrus* that contains the **premotor cortex**. On the inf. frontal gyrus identify **Broca's area** (motor speech area – within region of *inverse-shaped* □).

The **primary motor cortex** (Brodmann area A4) is the major source of fibres running in the corticospinal/corticonuclear tracts (60-70% of fibres). The remaining fibres (30-40%) originate from the **premotor** (A6) & **supplementary motor areas** (A8), and *primary somatosensory cortex* (see below). The corticospinal tract forms synapses on alpha-motor neurons and interneurons in ventral horn of the spinal cord, whereas the corticonuclear tracts innervates the cranial nerve nuclei. Most fibres of the corticospinal tract *cross in the pyramid* (*lat. corticospinal tract*), and the remaining fibres course *ipsilaterally* (*ant. corticospinal tract*).

The frontal motor cortical areas also innervate the **basal ganglia** and **cerebellum** (see neocerebellum). The *striatum* (caudate nucl. + putamen) is the origin of <u>direct</u> (cortex-striatum-internal pallidum-thalamus) and <u>indirect basal ganglia pathways</u> (cortex-striatum-external pallidum-subthalamic nucl.-internal pallidum-thalamus), inducing a disinhibition (activation by inhibition of inhibitory pathway) & inhibition of the thalamus, respectively. These pathways are under the modulatory control of the *substantia nigra (pars compacta)*, which sends dopaminergic fibres to the striatum. An activation of the direct pathway facilitates, and an activation of the indirect pathway inhibits movements. In *Parkinson's disease* the activity of the direct pathway is reduced resulting in akinesia / bradykinesia, and in *Huntington's disease* or *ballism* it is increased leading to hyperkinetic movements.

- <u>On the parietal lobe</u>, find the *postcentral gyrus* containing the **primary somatosensory cortex** located post. to the <u>central sulcus</u>. Discuss the somatotop organisation of this cortex, and identify the regions (limbs/trunk, head & neck) represented on *sensory homunculus*. At the post. end of the <u>lateral sulcus</u> find the *supramarginal* gyrus & *angular gyrus* (parieto-temporo-occipital junction).

The **primary somatosensory cortex** (Brodmann areas A3, A1 and A2) receives convergent input from the **posterior column pathway** [epicritic sensation for fine discriminative touch, vibration, limb position (proprioception), kinaesthesia and deep pressure], and **lateral spinothalamic pathway** (protopathic sensation for sharp, well-localised and fast temperature & pain). In both pathways the 1st order neuron is located in the *spinal ganglion*. However, the information in the <u>posterior column</u> pathway is relayed to the *ipsilat.* **cuneate & gracile nuclei** (brainstem), and from there over the *contralat.* thalamus (ventr. posterolat. nucl.=VPL; *med. lemniscus <u>crosses in brainstem</u>*) to the postcentral gyrus. In the <u>lat. spinothalamic pathway,</u> however, the 2nd order neuron in the dorsal horn projects via the *contralat.* spinal cord (<u>*crossing in spinal cord*</u>) and brainstem to the thalamus (VPL) and cortex. **Trigeminal fibres** from the **principal & mesencephalic sensory nuclei** transmit proprioception and touch (epicritic sensation), whereas fibres from the **spinal nucleus** of the trigeminal nerve relay pain and temperature (protopathic sensation). Both pathways cross in the brainstem, converge on the same thalamic nucl. (ventr. posteromed. nucl.=VPM), and terminate in the primary somatosensory cortex. Parietal lesions can induce *neglect* (ignoring body side), *apraxia* (inability to plan sequence of motor actions) & agnosia (disturbed recognition), **angular gyrus** lesions alexia (reading ↓), agraphia (writing ↓) & acalculia (calculating ↓).

- On the temporal lobe, find first the *sup., middle & inf. frontal gyri*. Now reflect the temporal lobe gently downwards with a tweezers to view the sup. temporal surface. Here you will see one or two (ant. & post.) *transverse gyri* or **Heschl's gyri** containing the **primary auditory cortex** (in right-handed person two gyri on the lt. & one gyrus on the rt.) that is surrounded by *secondary auditory cortex*. The region ant. to the transverse gyri is the *planum polare*, post. to it the *planum temporale* (contains Wernicke's area A22).

The **primary auditory cortex** receives *tonotopic* input from acoustic pathways originating in the inner ear (organ of Corti, spiral ganglion), which is relayed over the cochlear nuclei/ superior olivary complex, nuclei of lateral lemnisci, inferior colliculus and medial geniculate body to the **Heschl's gyri** (A41).
Lesion of the *left Brodmann area A22* on the *planum temporale* lead to **Wernicke aphasia** (comprehension of words severely impaired despite fluent speech, irrelevant words intrude) in a right-handed person. In contrast, a lesion of the *left A44* on the *inf. frontal gyrus* results in **Broca aphasia** (planning of motor speech disturbed, non-fluent < four words), agrammatism and paraphasic errors. Lesions is on the corresponding right A22 and A44 affect prosody (speech intonation).

- **Inspection of insula (lat. view)**
The insula is covered by extensions of the frontal, parietal and temporal lobes called opercula. Thus, the insula is connected to the three lobes through the **frontal, parietal & temporal operculum**. Therefore the insula can only be viewed in a specimen, if the three opercula have been removed:
- Identify the <u>central sulcus of the insula</u>. Posterior to this sulcus you will see the *long gyri of insula* (usually two gyri), and anterior to it the *short gyri of insula (4-5 gyri)*. The *limen insulae* is a small region connecting the insula anteriorly to the frontal lobe.

The insula receives input from the **spinothalamic pain and temperature pathways** (spinal ganglion neurons synapsing on ipsilat. dors. horn neurons, which send axons crossing in the spinal commissure & targeting the contralat. thalamus (ventral medial posterior nucleus VMpo). The thalamus then innervates the insula. In addition, the insula (and frontal operculum) receives input from **taste pathways** (taste buds on tongue and pharynx / larynx relayed by the CN. VII, IX and X to nucleus of solitary tract, and from there over pontine parabrachial nuclei to the thalamus and insula). The insula also contributes to the autonomic motor control of visceral organs (e.g. changes in heart rate, gastric motility).

- **Overview of telencephalon (med. view)**
- Above the corpus callosum, first identify the **cingulate gyrus** (part of the limbic lobe) below the <u>cingulate sulcus</u>.
- Next find above the <u>cingulate sulcus</u> the *sup. frontal gyrus* (frontal lobe) separated from the *paracentral gyrus* by the <u>paracentral sulcus</u>. The two parts of

the paracentral gyrus on the frontal & parietal lobes are separated by the medial extension of the <u>central sulcus</u> (difficult to distinguish on coronal sections).

- The precuneus (parietal lobe) is separated by the <u>marginal sulcus</u> from the paracentral gyrus, and by the <u>parietooccipital sulcus</u> from the cuneus (occipital lobe). On the occipital lobe also identify the **calcarine sulcus** and the **primary visual cortex** around the sulcus.

The **optic nerve** arises from retinal ganglion neurons (3rd neuron in *retino-geniculo-calcarine pathway*, see **Histology** for 1st-3rd order neurons & structure of retina). The 4th neuron in the pathway is located in the *lateral geniculate body*, and the 5th neuron in the **primary visual cortex** (**Brodmann area A17**). Fibres of the optic nerve coming from the nasal halves of the retina (rt. & lt. temporal visual fields) cross in the **optic chiasm**, whereas fibres from the temporal halves of the retina (rt & lt. nasal visual fields) stay ipsilaterally. The crossing and non-crossing fibres arriving from homonymous visual fields run together in the optic tract.

- **Overview of telencephalon and other basal structures (inf. view)**
In the inferior view, we will see structures in the di-, mes- & telencephalon.
- In the telencephalon inspect in the **frontal lobe** the *straight gyrus* separated from the *orbital gyri* by the <u>olfactory sulcus</u>. In the **temporal lobe** find the *temporal pole*, and then in medio-lateral direction the **parahippocampal gyrus** and its posterior extension called *med. occipitotemporal gyrus*. The <u>collateral sulcus</u> separates both gyri from the *lat. occipitotemporal gyrus* with the <u>occipitotemporal sulcus</u> at its lateral border.

The *cingulate & parahippocampal gyri* from an arch at the medial surface of the brain called **limbic system**, and are connected through the **Papez circuit**. In the modified (updated) Papez circuit, the entorhinal cortex on the ant. parahippo-campal gyrus (part of hippocampal formation in the broadest sense) provides input to the dentate gyrus and hippocampal sectors. The subiculum (part of hippocampal formation) provides hippocampal output to the hypothalamus (mammillary bodies), which in turn is connected through the thalamus (ant. thalamic nuclei) to the cingulate cortex (retrosplenial, anterogenual areas). The latter cortical areas innervate the entorhinal cortex closing the circuit.

- In the basal forebrain view the *olfactory tract*, and if present, also the **olfactory bulb**. At the *olfactory trigone*, the olfactory tract divides into the *med., intermediate and lat. olfactory striae*. Also view the optic nerves, chiasm & tracts, and lateral to the optic chiasm the ant. perforated substance.
- At the level of the optic chiasm find the *infundibular stalk*, and if present in the specimen, the *hypophysis*. Posterior to the optic chiasm find the mammillary bodies (hypothalamus) and the post. perforated substance.
- More posteriorly find the brainstem (mesencephalon) with the neighbouring med. & lat. geniculate bodies (metathalamus).

Olfactory fibres (CN. I) project directly to the *olfactory bulb* (see **Histology**) without running through the thalamus. The olfactory tract (contains ant. olfactory nucl. in primates) arises in the olfactory bulb. It innervates basal forebrain areas (e.g. olfactory tubercle, diagonal band) and divides at the olfactory trigone into the *med./intermediate* (to hypothalamus and habenula for subcortical activation of food intake & salivation) & *lat. olfactory striae* (to piriform cortex & other olfactory cortical regions influencing emotional learning).

- **Horizontal sections through internal capsule**

Here we will identify the fibre tract running through different subregions of the internal capsule:

- Find the **crus ant.** with the *frontopontine tract* and *ant. thalamic radiations*,
- the **genu** with the corticonuclear tract (motor nuclei of CN. III, IV, VI, V3, VII, IX-XI),
- and **crus post.** with the *corticospinal* (upper limb, trunk, lower limb in ant.-post. direction), *temporoparietopontine*, *corticoreticular*, *corticorubral* and *corticothalamic/thalamocortical tracts*.

The **cerebral cortex** has areas classified as allocortex, proisocortex and isocortex. The latter cortex has six-layers with a superficial molecular external granular, external pyramidal, internal granular, internal pyramidal and multiform layer (for further details see **Histology**). *Sensory cortical areas* have a broad *internal granular layer* (layer IV) and are called granular cortex, whereas *motor cortical areas* have a prominent internal pyramidal layer (layer IV), and in some areas even lack layer IV (agranular cortex).

NOTE: This practical should be also used to revise the neuronal systems mentioned above, but other pathways can also be discussed.

For example, *vestibular information* is relayed from the semicircular ducts (ampulla) and vestibule (utricle, saccule) over the vestibular ganglion (inner ear) to brainstem vestibular nuclei, which project to the oculomotor centres in the brainstem, cerebellum (particularly strong to vermis), and spinal cord (medial vestibulospinal tract to axial muscles, lateral vestibulospinal tract to limb muscles for skilled movements). Note that vestibular symptoms like vertigo & dizziness can be also found in temporomandibular joint (TMJ) disorders.

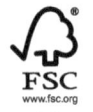